GW01466132

ANOTHER SPRING

M. D.

MINERVA PRESS
LONDON
MONTREUX   LOS ANGELES   SYDNEY

ANOTHER SPRING
Copyright © M D. 1997

All Rights Reserved

No part of this book may be reproduced in any form.
by photocopying or by any electronic or mechanical means.
including information storage or retrieval systems.
without permission in writing from both the copyright owner
and the publisher of this book.

ISBN 1 86106 277 X

First Published 1997 by
MINERVA PRESS
195 Knightsbridge
London SW7 1RE

Printed in Great Britain by
B.W.D. Ltd, Northolt, Middlesex

ANOTHER SPRING

For Tiger and Soldier

Foreword

On Monday, 25th January 1993 I woke up at eight fifteen. I felt bright and positive. This is not my normal way first thing in the morning and I attributed it to the new tablets I had been prescribed a couple of days before. As I sat on my bed with my cup of tea and smoking my start-of-day cigarette I knew what I had to do. It was still less then two months since this new episode in my life had begun, but I was all right. I felt I should record it for the sake of any others who find themselves in the same position, to encourage them and to show that it is not the end even though it may often feel like it. I've made no attempt to glamorise it, but there has been a lot that is new, that has been worthwhile and I have just told my story the way it happened, the way I experienced it. It has caused much soul-searching as I have endeavoured to come to terms with everything and to understand the people around me and the way they have reacted.

Part One

I am forty-one years old and by the time you read this I may be dead, for that is the point of this story. Or else this account will have been perhaps superfluous and there will be some pharmaceutical company laughing all the way to the bank. (Good luck to them, they would have saved my life.) I am a loner though I do have a handful of friends of whom I am very fond. I have a seventy-five year old mother and an unmarried sister who lives alone. I am very determined, but probably know when I am ultimately beaten.

I had always resolved not to test unless I felt I needed to. I had managed to save a little money and I imagined that if I tested positive it might change me. I thought I might go out and buy a Mercedes Benz or a Jag. Cars have always been a passion of mine and I would love to drive a big six-cylinder job, but my Polo was a far more suitable vehicle for the type of driving I did.

I had been losing weight probably since the beginning of the year. I attributed this to the fact that I was doing too much at work, the school meals had become dreadfully poor and at weekends, when I wasn't attending to everyday chores, I was dashing down to Surrey to see my mum. I had seen my doctor in the summer and confirmed more weight loss. I am 6' 1" and quite slim. I had lost a stone in weight and was now ten stone. I raised the question of testing with her, but I maintained that I did not believe that I had put myself at risk and decided not to.

Three months later I got a dose of flu. This always irritated me because I was the only person I knew who went along religiously each year in October to have a flu jab, I also seemed to be the only person who religiously each year in November got the flu. The first lot of antibiotics did not clear it up completely and so I went back to the doctor. I didn't feel that bad in myself except I had been feeling the cold. In fact, in the evenings in my uncentrally heated though certainly not unheated flat I had felt freezing cold. Also in the supermarket I found it almost unbearable to walk past the refrigerated display cabinets. This made it very difficult to select food.

So there I was again with my doctor, last appointment of the morning. We talked. She weighed me. I was horrified to see that I had again lost weight. Since the summer I had tried really hard to eat more and better. We talked some more and again I raised the question of testing. The Royal Free, I had thought, believing it to be the nearest place. I know there were tears in my eyes. Anyway Dr Segal – I like to give people names because they are real and important and each in his or her own way has helped me a great deal (In fact, lest I forget, I shall include my appreciation here. I have found people's kindness quite devastating, far more so than the knowledge of my infection or the prospect of my early death. The time in this first week which each granted me enabled me to come to terms just sufficiently to cope. I thank them all from the bottom of my heart.) – Dr Segal had heard that a unit had been opened in Northwick Park Hospital. This was, of course, much more convenient to me in Stanmore and therefore vastly preferable. She phoned them up and discovered that they had a clinic that afternoon.

On my way home I bought a hot pie in the cake shop. (These details seem important now, though I cannot actually remember what sort of a pie it was.) When I got back to the flat I put the pie in the bottom oven to make sure it was nice and hot. I realised then that the man (Kevin, I think) had come to resurface the roof garden. I had been waiting for this for about seven months and had been disappointed in the summer that I had not been able to grow any bedding plants, but I had imagined that the roof was about to be done and there had seemed no point. Anyway, I stuck my head round the patio door to say hello and to let him know that I had only popped in for about twenty minutes and was then off to an urgent appointment. I was really only hoping that he would let me eat my pie in peace and wouldn't expect a cup of coffee. I went back to the kitchen to get the pie and realised I had turned on the top oven so the pie had been sitting there getting cooler. I ate it, anyway. Kevin appeared, wanting something, I forget what.

So that afternoon, Monday 23rd November, I set off for Northwick Park Hospital. I found my way to the clinic without asking and walked into an immaculate new unit. I have not been to many hospitals, but those few I have visited have looked jaded. Discoloured or peeling paintwork, corridors damaged by hospital trolleys or beds being wheeled about. Perhaps the rest of Northwick Park is no better than those, but this clinic looked superb.

"I want to test for HIV," I said firmly to the receptionist. She was a coloured girl with a kind smile who could have been born for the job. This was Colette, as I discovered later. A form filled in and I was in the men's waiting room. It was very plush with its thick carpet, firmly upholstered green seats and a telly on a very hi-tech stand. There were all manner of leaflets on sexually transmitted diseases, and use of condoms as well as diet and exercise.

I think perhaps the lunchtime showing of *Neighbours* was on the box when I arrived, or it may have been *A Country Practice*. There was no one else in the waiting room and I did not have to wait long. I was shown to Karen's office, no bigger than a large cupboard, no window, but prettily decorated. Karen was the Health Adviser. I explained that because of my continuing weight loss I considered it necessary to test. Karen listened. I was tearful. I think I talked about my friend Howard who had died. I don't remember exactly, but I was with her for quite a while. Next the doctor, a sloppily dressed, though perhaps no less efficient for that, young woman took details of my medical history - nothing much to say, never ill. I never found out her name.

I used to hate going to the dentist until I changed my practice and discovered that there was a new school of dentistry, which was about twenty years more up-to-date where you were reclined .to the horizontal and where they had discarded the blunt old needles in favour of something which one scarcely felt at all.

Nonetheless, in my life I had only ever had two or three blood tests which I hadn't enjoyed, not because of the prick, but because I didn't like seeing a needle in my arm. I had always had to lie down. I am, every time, extremely apprehensive and I convey this apprehension to certain nurses and doctors and then things are prone to go wrong. Kathy, a somewhat older, kindly nurse, came in with the needle and I lay rigid on the bed, every vein defying her needle. And of course she missed the vein, or at least no blood came out. She would not try again, but fetched Anne whose needle recognised no such resistance. And then I chatted to Anne a bit. I talked about the test and how I had resolved not to test unless I thought it necessary. And then I broke down and cried for I realised inwardly that for me having the test signified that I was positive. There was no possible doubt. Kathy brought me tea, weak and sweet, just the way I like it, and they looked after me and mopped me up.

I went back to Karen who told me that I could have the result in a week. I looked at her forlornly and she said that she would ring up pathology on Wednesday morning to see if she could get the result by Wednesday afternoon.

I had, if it is possible, two best friends: Howard and Julian. I had met Howard when I was twenty-eight and Julian a couple of years later. Chalk and cheese these two. Howard thought Julian was boring and Julian probably thought that Howard was a lunatic, though he never would have said so. I needed them both for they reflected the different sides of my nature. About six or seven years ago Howard went on holiday with his parents to America. His father was giving a talk, as he did from time to time, to an assembled group of interested people, on aircraft windscreens. One evening, Howard, growing tired of the family room they were all sharing, went out on the town, met someone, went back, had a few drinks and stayed over, I think. On his return to England he was unwell. A year or so later at the insistence of a girl he was with whose name I shan't mention because I did not particularly care for her, he went to test and so did she. He was positive, she negative. Thank the Lord for the latter or else one would never have heard the end of it. Two years ago Howard died.

For the last ten years or so Julian has come round to my flat for a drink every Friday night. He is a person who sets great store by routine and I do not mean to diminish him in any way by that comment. We all adhere to certain routines in life. On the dot of eight o'clock Julian arrives and we have a mug of rather nice filter coffee which I have prepared. We talk about cars, computers, all sorts of things. At nine o'clock we watch the news. Then I clear the coffee things away and fetch the wine. We used to get through two bottles, but I found this too much so we reduced this to one bottle of one litre and we are now down to a regular bottle. We talk and at eleven o'clock he goes home. As he lives with his parents I am not allowed to ring him at home, and so every Wednesday evening between eight and eight thirty, without fail, he phones me from a public call box. We have a chat and every Wednesday evening I invite him round for Friday without which invitation I am sure he would not come.

That Monday evening, probably the only Monday evening ever, Julian rang. I forget why, it was certainly nothing very important. So I told him what I had done. He said I had been brave and that he would ring me on Wednesday. To me it had not been bravery it had been necessity, the time had come.

On Tuesday afternoon I went along to Edgware Chest Clinic to have an X-ray as Dr Segal had suggested, and then drove down to Temple Fortune.

When I was twenty I remember discussing psychoanalysis with an Italian lecturer that I had. It aroused my curiosity and interest sufficiently that I made it my business to find someone to go and see: Eva. Believing I had hit on an original woman I phoned up and made an appointment. I only saw her a couple of times. It was not practical. She was in Temple Fortune and I was two hundred miles away in Aberystwyth. But some years later when I started my job in Hertfordshire as a schoolteacher I returned to her and have seen her once or sometimes twice a week ever since. Tuesday five-thirty had become my regular spot.

I popped into WH Smith and bought a desk diary for my sister as I do every year. Over the road in Marks and Spencer I got her some marzipan fruits and I bought a box of chocolates for my mother. Apart from my Christmas cards, which some years ago I included in a database on the computer and which normally went out on 1st December each year (I am very proud of this system), I am not good at Christmas. This is because I do not like to shop. I am overpowered by the range of goods and don't know where to start; on some occasions I feel almost intimidated as the products sit there on the shelves, and in competition one with another seem to be shouting out: 'Buy me, buy me'. I am the sort of person who, at five o'clock on Christmas Eve, is still looking for the last one or two remaining and elusive presents. So it was quite out of character to have started my Christmas shopping in November.

At five thirty, sitting in the upstairs consulting room, I announced: "I am HIV positive, I have tested and I know that I am. I get the results tomorrow." Eva listened. She was surprised. I had rung her up on Sunday, which was unusual, and just said: "I don't feel well." We had talked a bit and, knowing my concern, she had said that I should test so that I could get on with my life. I had reasserted my intention not to, Eva listened and thought and finally said that I might have TB. Meanwhile I had already started winding my life down.

When a hospital rings you up at twenty to eight in the morning to invite you to attend the chest clinic at ten o'clock that same morning (presumably their first appointment) you know you've got problems. Well, at least they hadn't sent the hearse round. Apart from Dr Segal, who will always be young, most doctors seem middle-aged. This may have something to do with their white coats and their consulting rooms. At ten o'clock prompt, having been weighed by a nurse, I entered Dr Bradley's consulting room. Why is it that during the normal course of my life I have seldom met such warm, intelligent people as I was going to meet in the next few weeks? Dr Bradley is not one to beat about the bush. There were my two X-rays illuminated against the wall and I was told I had a small shadow, it was pointed out to me. I looked and saw a little white patch at the top of the left lung. I looked at her and said I didn't think it looked too bad and pointed out a nasty dark bit on the other X-ray, which I said I thought looked worse. Apparently we all have the nasty dark bits and a shadow on the lung is not, as I had imagined, dark but light. She said she thought I had TB. I sat and thought. Grasping at straws now I asked directly if she thought that the problem on the lung could be the cause of my weight loss or if she thought it was AIDS-related. She was very clear in her reply that she considered it the latter. We sat for some twenty minutes and talked about death and things. She did not hold out any false hope and I thank her for that.

As I sat there in tears (the last for a long time) she told me that she had lost her brother when he was only seventeen from asthma. She pointed out to me that I had opportunities now of which some people through sudden, unexpected death were deprived, basically to sort things out. I had the time to make a will, to tell people that I loved how I felt. But somehow it was the confidences that she shared with me that helped the most; her brother's death, the strange fact that she had always wanted to dye her hair green, her pride in her nails - she had suffered from anaemia and now, for the first time since an operation, she was able to grow them long. How she managed to introduce these last two items into our conversation seems a bit of a mystery now. I think perhaps we were just sharing secrets. She knew something about me and she was giving me something of herself in return.

Having explained my position regarding Northwick Park and my appointment that afternoon I was given my X-rays and off I went.

It was Karen's job to break the news to patients whether they were positive or negative, and what a dreadful job that must be, I thought. So at three thirty I went into her office, sat down and said, "Don't worry. I know. The doctor in Edgware told me this morning." I suppose I still hoped that Karen would say: "No, no you're wrong." Karen didn't say anything. She just looked at me - a long, kind look. In fact, no one has ever confirmed the result of that test for me and that is the way I want it left.

I told Karen I was afraid of dying. What I forget is that when you die you are not normally sitting up in a chair feeling as fit as I did chatting to someone. The body is failing, you are weary and perhaps even ready to let go. I was with my father as he died. He had battled with death for four weeks, but when the moment came I held one of his hands and my mother held the other, as with one long, long final exhalation he just stopped. I thought about this for a long time afterwards. If I had been told that I would be with my father when he died I would have been frightened, imagining he would do something; to die is after all a verb, but it describes the cessation of action. One should always be with those one loves as they die, it makes the grieving easier, I don't know why.

Next I was to see the doctor, in fact the consultant. His name was Kapembwa, but as most people couldn't say that, they called him by his first name, Moses. Karen told me. I always called him Dr Kapembwa and remember being quite irritated a couple of weeks later when my friend Lesley came to visit me in hospital and started talking about Moses, as if they were old pals. She had never met him, but knew someone who worked at St Mary's Hospital who had. I asked her to refer to him as Dr Kapembwa. Lesley was quite cross, but controlled her temper well. If I were being consulted by parents, I would not expect to be addressed as M. or, God forbid, mate.

He shook my hand firmly and looked me in the eyes. I returned his look. He spoke: "This is not a death sentence." I must admit I just thought to myself: 'Well, what is it?' Dr Kapembwa was right for me from the start. Here was a man who was wholly committed and sincere, a man I could trust with my life and would do so willingly. I just about managed to ask him if I would live till Christmas. I wanted to ask him if I would see another Spring, but I could not manage this. It was too emotionally charged. My father had died in March and at the time I remember hoping that he would see the Spring flowers a last time. I suppose he didn't, because he was in a hospital ward although we did have an unusually mild and sunny February that year (1988) which brought things on. The trittoleia had always been his favourites. Dr Kapembwa talked to me and looked at my X-rays. He confirmed Dr Bradley's opinion that I had TB. He would like me to come into hospital for tests and treatment for just a few days, maybe a week. TB is infectious, but only for a further five days after the beginning of treatment. He brought no pressure to bear on me. He told me to go home and think about it and to ring Karen the next day. I knew he wanted me to come in, I knew I would go.

The traffic in the Kenton Road is always dreadful in the rush hour and as I queued patiently I was planning. What did I need? Cigarettes, gin to fortify me. I drove straight to Safeway's and bought them. Time was getting on when I got back home. After a quick snack I got my case out and started to pack. What did one need in hospital? I didn't know. I packed as if I were going on holiday, leaving out the short-sleeved shirts and the swimming trunks. I waited quite some time for Julian's phone call. It came just before eight thirty, I confirmed my test result. Poor Julian, he hadn't slept a wink on Monday night. I rang my colleague, Maria, to tell her I was going into hospital and that the school could not expect me in for a while. That just left my mum and my sister. First I resolved that there would be no mention of HIV at this stage; it would be enough shock for them to hear I was going into hospital. In a very calm, reassuring voice I broke the news, I invited them both to ring me back later, which they did. I was worn out by now and still wanted to have a bath. I sat and remembered that *The Golden Girls* were on television. It had been Howard's favourite. I watched it. I had my bath. I had another gin and tonic and went to bed. I could not get off to sleep that night, but that was the fault of the gin.

The next morning I got up, washed and had a leisurely breakfast. Then I phoned the hospital and spoke to Karen. Yes, I would like to come in. She told me to come along to the clinic when I was ready. If I could make it for lunchtime that would be fine. Now again the pressure had been taken off me. I drove up the road to get some money. I had used up what I had on the cigarettes and gin. I bought *The Radio Times* and seven packets of Tunes. I was worried that they might not let me smoke. I was back home by ten thirty and booked a taxi for twelve o'clock. I was all ready to go. I sat and drank coffee, two cups maybe three. I felt surprisingly intact.

I got to the clinic with my heavy case and holdall and saw Karen. Dr Kapembwa was to examine me in the clinic before Karen took me up to the ward. I was anxious about two things only. Would they let me smoke? Could I have a room to myself? I explained that I had smoked twenty cigarettes at day for the last twenty years, that I was a committed smoker. Karen said she would have a word with the nurse, but thought it would be all right. And yes, I would have a single room. When I thought about it later this was pretty obvious you can't very well put someone who is infectious with TB into a ward with other patients.

There was quite a lot of hanging around that afternoon and I missed my lunch. First was Dr Kapembwa's examination; I confirmed my initial opinion of him. I think that a part of me perceived him as a father figure. I missed my own father enormously and he made me feel safe. He also had a sense of humour and said daft things to me while he examined me which made me laugh and feel generally comfortable with him. It was quite an examination, literally head to toe. He asked me questions about my body. Unfortunately I have kept a mental note of these and hence am aware of problems I may encounter as the infection progresses.

It must have been nearly five o'clock when Karen took me to the ward. Clarke Ward in the Lister unit, which was the isolation unit, must have been nearly half a mile away. That hospital is truly enormous. It was a nice little room that I had. It was about eleven foot square and one whole wall was a window which overlooked a car park. There was a little bathroom with toilet, handbasin and shower. In the room itself were a comfortable blue plastic armchair and one of those tables on wheels which you can raise so that you can eat your meals in bed. There was a locker with a television on it. This was fine. I would be all right here. In fact I can recall several hotel bedrooms from my childhood which did not measure up to this. I sat down in the armchair and had a cigarette, thus establishing myself. A nurse put her head round the door and saw that I was smoking. She disconnected the oxygen. "Don't want to blow the place up, do we?"

Before I had been able to unpack my things another doctor came in. She was much younger than me and very smart and proper. For the next two weeks Andrea was the doctor on the ward. She also examined me from head to toe. I suppose she went away and compared notes with Dr Kapembwa. They both had had a strange looking tool, like a very thin mallet with a circular end. They had only used it to test my reflexes, but I took a dislike to it.

Nothing had been ordered for me to eat that evening, but they had a spare vegetarian meal and so I had that. It was very good. Then I unpacked my things, sorted myself out and rang my sister and my mum to let them know I was comfortable. I was tired and I slept tolerably well.

There were two routines: the hospital routine and my own. Breakfast at ten past eight. Lunch at ten to twelve. Tea at ten to six. Each meal was followed by a cup of tea. There were in addition cups of tea at ten o'clock and three and a hot drink at half past nine, I had chocolate. During the morning the nurses came to strip and change my bed each day and at half past one a lady came in and washed the floor, dusted and cleaned the bathroom. Very often we ended up watching *Neighbours* together. My routine centred mainly around certain news broadcasts and programmes on radio and television. I listened to the end of the *Today* programme when I woke up. Then I washed, cleaned my teeth and put my clothes on. I always got washed and dressed no matter how long it took me. I had little rests. One morning it took me until midday. Another morning, when my temperature must have been quite high, I ran out of steam and called the nurse who helped me into my clothes. At ten thirty there was *Woman's Hour*. I watched the one o'clock, six o'clock and, if I could bear it, the nine o'clock news as well. In the afternoon, if there was a play on, I would start listening to it, but within three or four minutes I was invariably asleep. I found Radio Three a disappointment. I wanted to listen to familiar music - Mozart, Beethoven, Schubert. I hadn't even heard of most of the composers that were on offer and so I listened to Classic FM. In the evening I lay in bed listening to *The World Tonight*. By then I was tired and couldn't really follow what was being said about Bosnia or the fall of the pound, but I found the voices a comfort. Mostly I fell asleep with the radio still on and much later, after midnight, when broadcasting ceased and was replaced by a hiss, I dreamt that I was at home and no matter how I tried I could not turn the radio off. I pressed every button and turned every dial but all to no avail. Sometimes I would then wake up and switch it off. Sometimes it would go all night. These two routines helped me through the days which otherwise would have seemed quite lonely. There was always a cup of tea just round the corner or Moira Stuart's husky tones to look forward to.

There were two ward doctors: Andrea, who looked after me for the first two weeks, and then Juliet. They would regularly appear in my room with little trays containing syringes to take my blood. How were my electrolytes today? After the first two weeks when Andrea didn't appear I imagined she must be having a little holiday, and I envisaged her lying maybe on a beach somewhere with her little tray and her syringe beside her. Juliet, a very gentle, quiet girl, was just as bad. The day before I left the hospital she said she would come in to see me the following day to see if I had any final questions. The morning passed and there was no sign of Juliet. I was being fetched at two o'clock. Then at half past one she appeared and we chatted. I remember I was in tears of gratitude. Then, just as I thought she was about to leave she whipped out her little tray and syringe. I think I laughed out loud.

Apart from Andrea and Juliet there was a team of three doctors from the clinic. As well as Dr Kapembwa, whose patient I was and who saw me very frequently, there were Professor Pasvol and Dr Davidson. Every Thursday around lunchtime, and very often just as I was tucking into my lunch there was the so called grand tour. Dr Kapembwa was always there, together with either Andrea or Juliet and, it seemed to me, anyone else who was at a loose end and wanted to tag along. They were friendly and talked to me and made me feel important. They did not talk about me as if I wasn't there as I had seen happening in other hospitals where my father had been. What they said about me when they had left was another matter!

All the regular nurses were very kind to me and some also brought me a great deal of affection. If I have to return to hospital at a later stage I shall look forward to seeing them all. There were two in particular who spent a lot of time with me: Maggi and Freda.

Maggi has already moved on to promotion in another hospital. She was a very bright and cheerful girl who clearly intended concentrating her career on nursing HIV patients. When I had problems with one of the intravenous drugs it was she who suggested diluting it in a larger quantity of saline, which cured the problem. It was Maggi who came into my room one morning and said that she was taking me for a cup of coffee in the staff canteen that afternoon. It was quite a long walk through the hospital and my sense of achievement was enormous. I would have liked Maggi to have been on every day. Clearly this wasn't possible, but I missed her when she wasn't there. I later discovered that she had been working in St Mary's a couple of years before and had nursed Howard.

At night there was Freda. I first met Freda when the canula in my arm for the intravenous drugs packed up. I hadn't realised that canulas had to be moved from time to time. In my case it was every two days. I was very upset. She came back later that night to see that I was all right and we had a chat. Subsequent nights, when she had done her round, for she seemed to do all the IV's, she would come back to my room and, if I was still awake, she would come in and we would discuss things.

I must also mention Sue, who would always give me a hug and a kiss and who was so gentle with the IV drugs that I hardly ever felt a thing. Some evenings, however, it seemed as if there were no familiar faces. Whether through absence or short staffing there were times when it seemed as if the agency nurses took over. They were only there for a single shift and I suppose that they could not be expected to care in the same way the regular nurses did. I also thought that some of them were rather strange people.

The tea ladies also played an important part. They were, I suppose, quite lowly people. They were mainly middle-aged, some quite pretty. Some spoke to me, others didn't. Perhaps they didn't know English apart from to ask: "Cup of tea?" and to understand my reply: "Oh, yes, please," which I always said with a great enthusiasm, which I felt. Perhaps my tastes changed with the drugs I was taking, but the tea seemed to get sweeter and sweeter. Later on, when I was recovering, and I took a walk down the ward and passed the tea trolley, I noticed they were using a dessert spoon for the sugar.

Initially I received few visitors. Not many people knew I was in hospital, Julian came. I felt so sorry for him the first time. He wouldn't remove his anorak, and sat in the considerable heat in my room dressed for the outside with a transparent apron, a face mask and the disposable rubber gloves which were the requirement for visiting me, suspected as I was of having TB. On later visits he risked removing his outer clothing and looked more comfortable. My mum came too. She had a dreadful drive up to the hospital, coming as she was from Leatherhead. It is one of the most tedious drives I know through the outskirts of London the whole way. I was always concerned for her because, quite apart from the drive, I knew how worried she was about me. Later on she started to use public transport.

Then there were colleagues from work who began to visit. I became increasingly anxious lest hordes of people started to turn up. I have worked in the same place for about seventeen years and know most people there, a staff of about seventy, quite well; I was keen to restrict the visiting to the handful of colleagues with whom I had had a genuine rapport in the past, and so I got Maria to put it about at work that I was too ill to be visited. This was a lie. Visiting was also to be restricted to one at a time. This was my rule. If people wanted to visit me they should come and have a conversation with me. I did not like the idea of people coming and sitting in my room and talking to one another or possibly even laughing and joking. Mike and Mike were the one exception that I made.

Maria, Viva and Wendy came from work and my assistant Sandra, who, in the meantime, had leapt into my administrative job. I was quite pleased for her and felt that it was I who had enabled her to take over. I told Maria, Viva and Wendy about the HIV; I knew I could count on them.

Then, on the second Sunday my mother came up by car in the morning and left just after I had had my lunch. In fact, when she was visiting I always used to order a bowl of soup with my lunch so that she could have something to eat. Twenty minutes later she was back with my sister. Now she lives two hundred miles away in the North. She was the last person I was expecting to see though I was looking forward to seeing her at Christmas. I was quite overwhelmed and burst into tears. I wanted to give her a hug, but as always I was only offered the side of her forehead to kiss and a comment such as 'Don't be so silly'. This took the wind out of my sails, but I felt sorry for her, unable as she was to accept this spontaneous gesture of affection.

There were, however, other friends, quite dear friends who didn't know where I was. I felt a peculiar reluctance to phone and so it wasn't until the second week that I rang Lesley, Health Adviser for HIV and AIDS and condom expert, the third week that I rang Peter, badminton partner and friend, and the last week that I got in touch with Mike and Mike, friends who had lived in the same block of flats with me. They all came bearing gifts - chocolate, toffees, biscuits, jam, wine, grapes, fruit, pot plants, Christmas trees (I had two), cuddly toys and cigarettes. Apart from the cigarettes and Smarties that Julian brought me I did not want any of these things. I had gone off chocolate and sweet things, but I did still enjoy the Smarties which I ate one at a time as I lay in bed at night listening to the radio. It seems now that it was ungrateful on my part, but I had nowhere to put these things. I tried stowing them in my case, but later on when I became ill I was too weak to burrow under them to get fresh clothes out of my case and gave up changing my clothes altogether. My mother, realising my frustration, gave all these things to the nurses. They were pleased and I had my space back again.

The first few days after I had settled in I felt pretty good. Visitors were surprised that I was up and dressed and probably seemed the same as ever. The doctors came daily to check on me. I was given a skin test to confirm that I had TB, but this turned out to be negative. Dr Kapembwa decided that I should have a bronchoscopy. I hadn't heard the word before, but I knew what it meant. He told me a few days in advance. I worried myself half to death about it, but better that than having it sprung on you. In the end Maggi said she would come down with me while it was being done.

Rob Wilkinson was the bronchoscopy man, a very nice man, I was told, and Mondays and Wednesdays were the days he performed his skill. And so from midnight on Tuesday, 1st December it was NIL BY MOUTH. I asked if I could have just a cup of tea and a fag the next morning and received a decisive "No" in reply. I had the pre-med and was wheeled off in my bed. I suppose I had imagined that after the pre-med I would feel barely alive. This was not the case, so when I saw Dr Wilkinson I told him I wanted a shot in the arm. He gave me one. I had to snort up an evil tasting gel through one nostril so that it started running down the back of my mouth. This anaesthetised the passage. Rob was into my lung in a flash and taking his washings. It seemed to be over very quickly and I had felt nothing at all. A skilled operator indeed. I felt proud, felt I should have been given a badge.

Unfortunately, that afternoon I had two visitors. I say unfortunately because instead of sleeping off the pre-med and resting after the morning's procedure I sat up in bed and chatted. I did not feel good that night and my temperature was high. The following day my temperature was higher still and Dr Kapembwa decided it was time to act. The washings from the bronchoscopy had revealed nothing. I could hear Dr Kapembwa and Andrea discussing me outside my door. Dr Kapembwa was saying: "What we are dealing with here are probabilities." I thought, 'Great. They don't know what's wrong.'

I was put on intravenous antibiotics. Two were squirted in from a syringe and the third was a drip. I found out later that this is known as a cocktail. I didn't mind the drip, but one of the other antibiotics irritated my vein and it wasn't very nice. I continued with these drugs over the weekend. However, my temperature did not come down and I was taken off the IV's. I was given another skin test, ten times the strength of the previous one. It too was negative.

I also had a CT chest scan. This was actually quite hard work having to hold my breath for ten seconds every minute or so; an older person would be quite exhausted.

Then Dr Kapembwa decided I should have a second bronchoscopy, this time with biopsy. Again I signed my consent. I didn't feel any braver about it than the week before. In fact I didn't manage quite as well. I imagine that this was because they used a slightly larger tube. I coughed a lot and apologised a lot. That afternoon I was wheeled down to X-ray. The shadow on my lung had completely vanished.

The next day Dr Kapembwa appeared. They had got the bug. It was pneumonia. I was put back on the drip with another antibiotic, Septrin. They decided to give me some blood that weekend, four units. By Sunday my temperature was back to normal. On the Monday I was taken off the drip and the medication continued orally. I felt pretty darned good. On Tuesday, when Mike and Mike visited, we drove into Harrow for a cup of coffee.

Then on Wednesday while I was eating my lunch and looking out over the car park I realised I didn't feel quite right. Was it my vision? I couldn't quite describe it. I had a rest that afternoon. On the

Thursday Dr Kapembwa said that he thought I could go home on Friday so long as I came back the following week to be checked. By the evening I could not walk ten steps. I was very upset and a bit frightened. I remember sitting on the edge of my bed with Maggi and saying that I couldn't go home like that. She agreed. I phoned my mum to delay my return. I told the doctors and everyone who came into my room that it was the Septrin that was making me feel so awful. I felt that they didn't believe me, but I knew it was. If I had managed it intravenously why should it cause me problems orally? I didn't know the answer to that, but I felt absolutely dreadful. My legs were failing, I was confused. I felt you could have wrung the medication out of my body. I felt drenched in it. They seemed to think that the problem was psychological, that I was depressed. I considered this; they were mistaken. On the Friday Dr Kapembwa stopped the Septrin and over the weekend it started very slowly to drain out of my body, though I didn't feel it had all disappeared for two more weeks. Very slowly my strength began to return.

The following Wednesday, two days before Christmas, I was discharged. I would miss my little room and the nurses.

During the first few days in hospital before I became ill I had a lot of time to think. It was less than a week since I had been tested and when, on the Wednesday afternoon I had asked Dr Kapembwa if I would live till Christmas it had been a serious question. I guess I was now hoping that if I could just hang in there, there might yet be another Spring. I was not looking beyond that. I knew that Howard had gone quickly. He was taken ill in June. I didn't know at the time. Despite our close friendship there could be quite long periods of time when we weren't in touch. I had sent him a birthday card, but didn't hear from him. I should have guessed. I didn't receive his letter until the beginning of August. It had no stamp on it. It was written in the same cheerful, light-hearted tone that was always Howard's nature, but I knew that he was telling me that he was ill and wanted to see me.

I went round to his house. He opened the door and I went into the hall. He just said to me, "I need a hug." As we hugged one another I thought to myself: 'Never forget this'. He put me to sit in the garden with a couple of magazines. He said he needed to rest. About an hour later he re-emerged, having been unable to sleep. We made a cup of tea and had some of his gran's sponge cake. Howard told me everything that had happened. He talked a long time about his illness. He showed me his hands; they were blue. He showed me the lesions on the insides of his upper arms. Then we went inside because he wanted to watch *Eastenders*. We decided to have a gin and tonic. Then his gran appeared with a cup of tea so we sat there with a gin and tonic in one hand and a cup of tea in the other. I always associate gin and tonic with Howard. Not that he drank much, but it was he who, many years before, had given me my first.

The next time I saw Howard he was in hospital, St Mary's. He looked all right to me and was sitting up in bed watching the television. We talked. I certainly didn't think he was at death's door. The following week I was on holiday. When I returned I went to visit him again. In the week I was away he had wasted away. He was terribly thin and weak. He could not now sit up in bed. I remember looking at his neck. It seemed no thicker than most people's arms. It was the last time I saw him. That weekend I went to visit my mother to celebrate my birthday, I think. We went out for a walk after lunch. She slipped, fell and broke her wrist and so I stayed to look after her. I phoned the hospital three times to get news of Howard. 'He was a little better.' 'No change'. 'He had died the previous day.'

I know that I said that I felt one should be with those one loves when they die, but I think it was perhaps a good thing I wasn't with Howard for I believe I would have howled my grief and anger through the streets like some mortally wounded animal. He was twenty-eight years old and he was my friend. My mother was reading the newspaper in the lounge on the morning that I rang the hospital the last time, and when I came in started telling me about a new drug (ddI).

I said, "It's too late for Howard."

My mum just said, "Poor lamb."

Some nights later I dreamt that Howard was going on a bus journey. He saw me, jumped off the bus to give me a kiss and nearly missed it - I wish he had.

At least I was forty-one and had had twenty or so years of adult life. At twenty-eight there is so much still to experience and to discover - both good and bad.

Sitting there in the hospital in those first few days I assumed that I didn't have long. There were things to be done, I made a list. I must write a will, I wanted to remember all my friends with some small amount of money, I must go and see the vicar. Although I had met him, when my father died, he didn't know anything about me. What music did I want to be played at my cremation? I must write a last letter to my sister and my mum which they could keep for ever and which should be a comfort to them.

I did write a couple of letters that first week, one to Dr Bradley thanking her for her kindness and assuring her that I was cared for, and another to Professor Prance. The first Sunday I had been listening to *Desert Island Discs* and Professor Prance, who is director of the Royal Botanic Gardens in Kew, was talking about important research projects which were currently being undertaken in the laboratories. He announced that they had found a cure for AIDS, which was at that moment undergoing clinical trials. The plant concerned was the Morton Bay Chestnut, which has powerful antiviral properties. My heart had leapt and I immediately wrote to him. I did get a reply about a month later. He had delegated this responsibility. I was advised to write to two addresses. It seemed that there were certain herbal formulations claimed to alleviate the symptoms. There was no more talk about a cure. I suppose it had been too good to be true. One would hardly announce the cure for AIDS on *Desert Island Discs*.

Then there was the ghastly job of telling my mother and my sister about the HIV. Both Karen and Dr Kapembwa had advised me to hold back before telling anyone I was HIV positive and to consider carefully first whom I wanted to know. They pointed out that once I had told someone, there was no going back. This was valuable advice because, before it, I had been in a frame of mind to have told everyone.

I am not ashamed, but it is not everyone's business and there are always those who would use it to their advantage or not be able to keep it to themselves.

I would have preferred to have told them when I saw them, but as my sister wasn't coming until Christmas and I didn't want to spoil Christmas with further bad news I had no option but to tell them over the phone. On the second Friday that I was in hospital someone announced on the radio that it was three weeks to Christmas; I knew that I had to tell them that day. It was important that it was a Friday so that Eleanor could at least begin to come to terms with it before she had to go back to work on Monday. I knew what it was like to be told. I remembered Howard telling me. For some reason which I do not understand it is far worse for those being told than for me who had the virus. I phoned my sister first and discussed with her whether I should tell my mum. Then I rang my mum. This was for me the hardest thing to do. I guess I was lucky, I knew that I would receive their unquestioning support and sympathy. Others are not this fortunate.

Then I thought about my job. I could see clearly now what I had known from the start, how wrong it was for me. I felt I had wasted seventeen years of my life there. Education and teaching weren't wrong for me, but that comprehensive school had very little to do with learning, it was a dreadful place. The children weren't stupid, but for the most part they weren't interested and didn't want to know. When the examination results were published last year for the first time it showed that our school was near the bottom of the list. Teachers struggled with discipline and were treated with contempt. The order of the day among many of the older children was to show off and swear constantly and to spit, which they called 'gobbing'. They covered door handles and banisters with spit. They stood at upstairs windows and spat at one another and teachers. I was only hit once, I was very upset, but knew not to take it personally. They lounged around in the classroom, doing as little as possible, continually making a nuisance of themselves and being abusive. Sometimes they would gang up against a teacher and make his life hell. Eventually, when they reached the fifth form and began to play truant, everyone was glad. At least I would never have to go back.

I spent ages wondering how I had become infected. I realised that this was a semi-futile occupation. On the one hand it changed nothing, but on the other it might give me an indication as to how long I had left. It seemed that looking back over the last ten years I had played it pretty safely. AIDS had hit the headlines in 1981. I had had a short-lived relationship in 1979 with someone who had travelled in the United States. It had knocked me for six. I had spent years getting over it. Both mentally and physically it had caused me problems. I remember telling my analyst I thought I had a virus in my brain. Since then there had been one other person, but I was unwilling to believe it was him. He was twenty-two and had only just come to the London area. Could it be that I had had this virus for thirteen years? I think I must have, but I will never know.

I recalled the relationships that I had had over the last twenty years. There were not many. I remembered the investment I had made in them and my pain each time when they ended. I felt no pain now, just a sadness that there was no one to whom I was physically close. I was not in touch with any of them anymore except for Clive. I had been happy with him, but I hadn't been in love and it had been partly my fault we had split up. I owed him an apology and now after fifteen years he would finally have it.

I felt most of all angry, very angry. I was angry with myself. I was angry that I had been stupid enough to contract this infection even though it may have been at a time before it was known of or even had a name. I was angry also that sex, which is meant to be pleasurable and fun could prove to be so deadly. And I was ready to fight. The battle lines were drawn up. The fight was on and I would never give up, ever.

Part Two

I arrived home about an hour after my sister, who had driven from the North. I fetched my holdall from the car boot and went into the lounge. I sat down in an armchair which I then adopted for the next few weeks as a replacement for the blue plastic one in the hospital. Was I glad to be home? It was nice to see my mother and sister, but I felt apprehensive. I had grown accustomed to my little room and the hospital routine. Would I be able to cope back at home? Cups of tea were made for me and cakes were offered to me which I gratefully consumed, and I just sat in that gold-coloured armchair which I found comfortable, and from where I could look around me at my new yet familiar surroundings.

I wasn't expected to do anything. In any case I couldn't have. Meals were in the dining room, and so with an effort of will I pushed myself out of my chair and made my way there. My appetite was excellent. I ate anything that was put my way. When I left the hospital I was only nine stone despite the fact that I had eaten everything I had been given. I had decided that it was crucial to my survival that I should put on weight, and I was prepared to eat a great deal to achieve this end.

I felt not so much weak as weary and this extreme weariness continued for some weeks. I was also very slow. I remember I had a bath that evening. It took me nearly an hour. When I got out I checked my weight. As I thought - nine stone. I said to myself that I still did not look ridiculously thin though when I was in the bath I could feel there was not much flesh on me and I had to be careful moving around in it in order not to hurt myself.

It was like a bad dream from which there was no waking. Each morning when I woke my first conscious thought was always: 'I am HIV positive.' I spent those first few days really just moving from my chair to the toilet or the dining room and, in the afternoon, sleeping. It was a very heavy sleep and I knew it wasn't a healthy sleep. The conversation in the house always returned to my illness as we all tried to understand it and come to terms with it.

Two days later it was Christmas Day. I had been looking forward to Christmas and to spending it quietly with just my mum and my sister. In the bathroom that morning as I was cleaning my teeth I thought to myself: 'This is my last ever Christmas.' We had a nice day, opening our presents in the morning after coffee. I had asked my mum to get me an electric blanket. I thought this would be useful in my chilly bedroom in Stanmore. My sister gave me a shirt. I enjoyed my lunch, I always do.

Then on the Sunday my mum encouraged me to come for a short walk. It was pretty cold, about four degrees, but I put my jacket and my anorak on and we walked up the road. It felt all right in the sun so we decided to carry on a bit further, in fact to do a circular walk. When we were about half-way the wind got up and we were out of the sunshine. I started feeling cold, desperately cold, but there was no point turning back now and so we strode on at a great pace. There was nothing wrong with my legs. I did think about knocking on the door of a house and asking to use the phone to get Eleanor to pick us up, but I don't like to give up. I was so relieved when we got back to the warmth of the house, I lay down on the sofa and fell fast asleep till lunchtime.

It was that evening also that after my bath I got on the scales again. I thought that, like Howard, I was wasting away and wanted to check whether my weight had fallen below nine stone. I looked and couldn't believe my eyes. I got off the scales to check the pointer was at zero and then got back on. Nine and a half stone. I sat on the stool in the bathroom and wept. For the last year I had just lost weight. Now I had suddenly put on half a stone and if I could put on half a stone in five days I could perhaps put on more. It felt like time for celebration. It certainly marked an upturn in my spirits and made me even more determined. Now I had something I could aspire to. I felt that if I could increase my weight I would improve my resistance to infection and so my chances of survival.

I had asked Eleanor to drive me up to Stanmore the next day. There were two reasons for this. The first was that I wanted to fetch my car. For me it is an important friend and I wanted it standing outside the house even if I wasn't using it, it would also enable me to drive up to the clinic for my appointment the following week myself, without having to depend on someone to drive me there, wait around and bring me back. The other reason was that I wanted to have some time to be totally alone. We set off with enough food for twenty-four hours and arrived at the flat. It looked the same as when I had left it. It was a bit dusty, but nothing like as bad as I would have imagined. We attached the electric blanket to the mattress and changed the bedding and then had lunch. Eleanor set off back and I was alone. I put the washing on and attended to a couple of bills which had come in my absence and then had a sleep. It was about five o'clock when I woke and I was feeling cold. I heated some soup to warm me up and then made an omelette. It was strange to be back in the flat. I like my flat, but I felt no affection for it or for my possessions. This surprised me. My affection was reserved for the people who had stood by me and come to visit me in hospital.

It was pretty tough being there on my own, particularly as it turned out to be such a cold night, minus five degrees. The electric blanket proved its value immediately. It seemed an unparalleled luxury.

The next morning, as always, I was very slow. I had to make my own breakfast and wash up. I had to wash myself and shave. I had to get dressed and I had to shut the flat up. All this took quite some time and I had to sit down and have a rest before I left. The car, which I had been worried about, started on the button. Driving was no problem, probably because I was sitting down, but I decided not to use the motorway just yet.

I got back home at about midday. I was very glad to be back and made my way immediately to my armchair in the lounge. The trip had fulfilled a need in me. I had fetched the car, I had seen the flat and I had been alone for a little while.

Thursday was New Year's Eve. I had brought back a half bottle of champagne from the flat. I had bought it in France the previous July when, accompanied by four other members of staff and fifty children, we had spent a day in Boulogne. Viva was expert in organising these trips. The only year she didn't it had been a complete disaster. The champagne had been intended for my birthday, but for some reason I hadn't drunk it. We were going to wait up until midnight, but as I thought it unlikely that I could possibly still be awake at that time and Eleanor, who in any case likes to hit the hay early, was driving back to the North the next day, we had it at a quarter past ten. I don't know that any of us really like champagne, but it seems to be the thing to do. We would probably all have preferred a cup of tea.

I suppose in some ways I was a little better than when I left hospital, but really I was sleepier and more weary than ever. I'd get up and have my breakfast, a bowl of porridge, a piece of toast and a cup of tea. I would wash up the bowl, the plate and the cup and saucer. I would go back upstairs and wash and shave before making for the chair in the lounge. This degree of activity wore me out and I would fall asleep. After lunch too I slept. It was only really in the evenings that I had a little more energy.

So the following week promised to be a hard week for me with four different appointments. For the last couple of years I had been seeing a skin specialist in Edgware hospital every three months. I had had problems initially with the skin on my face. My father had suffered severely from psoriasis and I assumed that I had inherited a mild form of this from him. In fact it was two conditions, psoriasis and folliculitis. However, by using hydrocortisone cream and a special shampoo it was well under control. In the hospital I had been given a little booklet published by the makers of the anti-viral drug AZT which mentioned dermatitis as a symptom of HIV infection. I had decided that it would be more sensible to transfer this treatment also to Northwick Park so that it would be all under one roof. Anyway I thought that I would attend my appointment in Edgware and tell Dr Robinson what I was doing and why. He was very nice to me. He confirmed that my skin condition could be caused by HIV. He took his time and talked to me. He didn't know quite what to say, but he tried hard and I knew he was wishing me well.

The following day, the Thursday, was the main appointment of the week when I was returning to the clinic. I was full of apprehension. I didn't really know why. Was it just anxiety about having my blood taken again? Was it fear that they might want to take me back into hospital? As I walked into the hospital entrance I became suddenly self-conscious. There were loads of people and I thought they might be looking at me and thinking to themselves: 'There's an ill person' or worse still 'There's a person with AIDS'. I knew that this was silly because despite my weight loss and being a bit thin in the face I looked all right and I was wearing a very nice jacket which seems to have become my constant companion since I became sick in November. It is a blue check and I am very attached to it.

I had a tremendous welcome from Colette when I walked into the clinic and later on from Anne and Kathy, the nurses. I sat down in the waiting room and Anne came to tell me that I was to be seen by Dr Davidson because Dr Kapembwa was on study leave. I swore blind that I didn't know a Dr Davidson. However, when I saw him I recognised him as one of the doctors who had accompanied Dr Kapembwa on the grand tour. He had also come to see me by himself one evening and we had talked about Armistead Maupin's *Tales of the City*. He asked me how I was and I told him I was tired. He seemed to assume that I was at work. Then he examined me, head to toe, as usual and said, "Physically you are one hundred per cent and you look a picture of health." We went to his consulting room and with no prompting from me he started me talking about my life expectancy. He said, "You may not live until you're ninety, but you could outlive me and I would expect you to live to see the millennium." Dr Davidson is quite a young man and I wasn't prepared for this and it was stored at the back of my mind to be dealt with later.

He started talking about AZT. I would have to decide whether I wanted to take it. When I had been in hospital also, every time AZT was mentioned it was inferred that I had a choice either to take it or not. I had read about it and knew the possible side-effects: headaches, vomiting in the short-term, anaemia requiring periodic blood transfusions in the long term. I was also under the impression that I had read somewhere that it turned the fingernails blue, but as I can no longer find reference to this I must assume that it was a particularly vivid dream that I had or that someone was pulling my leg. I said to Dr Davidson that I was aware of the possible side-effects, but, insofar as this was the drug which could prolong my life, I saw no possible reason for not taking it. I was so positive in my response that he said, "Well, we'll start today."

Anne took my blood, just half an armful, and I went down to the X-ray department to have a chest X-ray. I sneaked a look at it before returning with it to the clinic. The shadow had reappeared. Bugger. I gave the X-rays to Dr Davidson and went and had a chat with Karen. A while later he came and interrupted us. There was no sign of pneumonia on the X-rays. As for the shadow he thought it was probably nothing to worry about. Indeed he thought it might be something I had had for a long time. It could be a cyst which during the second bronchoscopy, as a result of my coughing, had discharged itself and had now filled up again. Not to worry. So I went home and took the first two tablets, I didn't tell anyone what Dr Davidson had said about living to see the millennium, but I slept badly that night.

The following morning I had arranged to see Eva at eleven o'clock. She opened the door and I walked in. She gave me a hug and I asked if I could have a cup of coffee. I started crying even before I got to the consulting room. She was still downstairs getting my coffee. I don't know precisely what the tears were saying, something like, 'I'm back despite everything.' I cut the tears short because there was so much I wanted to tell Eva. She had come to visit me in the hospital and I had been in touch by phone since, but I wanted to tell her about what Dr Davidson had said the day before. She seemed sceptical.

The last appointment of the week was with Dr Segal at five-thirty. Rousing myself from a fairly deep sleep I picked up my list of things to say and my discharge certificate from the hospital and made my way up the road. Here again I had a tremendous welcome. The appointments are only ten minutes, but I must have spent nearly half an hour with her. I felt sorry for the young man who was waiting.

She had rung the hospital while I was there, but wanted to know all about what had happened. As briefly as I could I told her about the bronchoscopies, the antibiotics, the problems with the Septrin and how I had now started on the AZT. She thumbed back through her notes on me and found that she had prescribed Septrin for me in 1982 and I had had no problems with it. She remembered also that in 1985 I had had pneumonia which had responded very readily to the antibiotics she had given me.

It was good to be back and seeing these people again. At eight o'clock Julian came round and we had our coffee and talked. Then I opened the wine, I only had two glasses, but it was a start. I sent him home at a quarter past ten.

The next day I returned to Surrey. I was very tired and relieved to let my mother see to the cooking and everything. It was around this time that I started reading. I picked up a book by PD James, *Devices and Desires*, a nice long book, and when I wasn't sleeping I read. I enjoyed it enormously and was very impressed by her skill as a writer. Other books followed: *Hotel du Lac*, *Emma*, *Love and War in the Apennines* and another by PD James. I have never been one to read for pleasure, I have always been a very active person, always doing things like swimming or playing sport.

As part of my degree course was German literature I had had to read a great deal at university, but the pleasure for me lay in studying and discussing texts. As a child I had read very little. The only book I remember was *The Silver Sword* which I had loved. Even now I can hear my father's voice saying to me: "Why don't you sit down and read a book?" Probably I was being particularly annoying at the time. Reading was a hobby I was reserving for my retirement, my old age when I wouldn't have the energy to be doing things the whole time. Probably this had been a mistake.

I was really worried that I might experience side-effects from the AZT and be unable to continue with it, but the days passed and I had no adverse reaction at all, no blue fingernails. Meanwhile I was continuing to put on weight. Every day I had a good lunch and a cooked tea; what's more I was enjoying the food and not overeating. I weighed myself once a week on Sunday and each time I had gained a pound or two. It looked like ten stone might be possible. As the weight went on, gradually my resistance to the cold began to increase though I still could not cope with an outside temperature of less than four degrees.

The weariness, however, continued unrelieved, I think I almost revelled in it. I enjoyed these little sleeps I had from which I sometimes awoke feeling quite disorientated. I would wake up suddenly feeling mildly anxious. Had I missed breakfast? No, it was five o'clock in the afternoon. Was tea ready? No, we hadn't had lunch yet. Yet the weariness did not prevent me from doing things I had to; I could pull myself together to drive to Stanmore, attend my appointments or do a bit of shopping, but when I returned either to the house or the flat I just slumped into a chair and slept. I didn't feel that the clinic had really appreciated how tired I was most of the time and I resolved that I must try to impress on them the full extent of this weariness.

It was Professor Pasvol that I saw the following week. I sat next to him trying to look at the long printout showing the results of the tests that had been made from my blood. It meant nothing to me. He looked at the printout and assumed that I was at work. It always made me feel guilty that I wasn't, but I told him about my tiredness. I had been told that the pneumonia might recur and knew that I would need prophylaxis to try to prevent this happening. It seemed that there were two drugs available, Septrin or Pentamidine. The Septrin was taken orally but the Pentamidine was inhaled once every four weeks using the nebuliser in the clinic. Professor Pasvol seemed to favour the Septrin and so, despite my bad experience with it in the hospital, I agreed. I said to myself that the prophylactic dose would be much lower than what I had been taking. When I got home I looked at the tablets. They were of course exactly the same as I had taken before and I was not looking forward to them. They are dispersed in water and drunk, it was quite the vilest thing I have ever tasted. Still it was only three times a week, Mondays, Wednesdays and Fridays, two tablets twice a day.

The next morning I got up and before doing anything else I had two tablets of Septrin. Get it over and done with, I thought. Perhaps it didn't taste quite as bad as I remembered. I had my breakfast and set off down to see Eva. On the way down I developed a headache. I went to the bank to get some money from the machine in the wall. It was raining a bit and I felt very cold. Eva got me some coffee and I carried on crying from the week before. It seemed cold in the consulting room and I started shivering. Eva gave me a blanket, but I could not warm up. After the session I got back in the car to drive home. With the heater full on I could barely control my feet to operate the pedals I was shivering so much. I walked into the flat and before I could take my anorak off I felt slightly nauseous. No sooner than I had had this thought than I started to vomit. I raced to the toilet. I was about three foot away as I aimed towards the toilet pan. I made it, thank God. I vomited three more times equally violently. Then, freezing cold, shuddering with my whole body and fully clothed I got into bed with the blanket on. I was frightened. The shuddering continued for over an hour. At two o'clock I decided to try to get up and ring the clinic. I think I really wanted them to send someone round to look after me, but of course I didn't say so. I spoke to Karen who said she would have a word with Dr Kapembwa and ring me back. She thought I could try to have a cup of tea. She was obviously busy that afternoon and I seemed to wait hours for her call. I sat there frozen, with a thumping head and time just seemed to have come to a standstill and wouldn't move on. In the end I rang back, but Karen wasn't there. Eventually she did ring. The doctors did not want me to give up the Septrin. They had to be joking.

I had invited Mike and Mike round that evening, I rang them up and told them how dreadful I was feeling but that I would still like them to come. I needed the comfort of other human company. When they arrived I was still sitting there in my jacket with the heating pumping out everything it had. It was good to see them. After a while Mike made me a piece of toast which I ate with honey and a mug of hot milk. At last I started to feel warmer and eventually I was even able to take my jacket off. I felt tired and so they left at about ten o'clock. I went to bed and listened to the radio until about eleven. When I awoke it was five past seven. Too early to get up. Twenty minutes later it was still five past seven. There was no sleep left in me so I got up and put the light on. It was in fact only one o'clock in the morning. I had been deceived by the alarm hand which still pointed to seven o'clock. I made a cup of tea. There wasn't much I could do. My head was still pounding so it wasn't worth putting my lenses in as reading was out of the question. I sat in the lounge drinking cups of tea until three o'clock when I went back to bed and lay there listening to Classic FM until five o'clock. I put the light out and slept until nine.

I was meant to be driving back to Surrey that day to see my uncle David, my father's step-brother, who was visiting from the States, but the episode with the Septrin had drained my last reserves of energy and I couldn't go. I phoned Lesley to ask her to get me a pint of milk. She brought it round in the afternoon and stayed a couple of hours. She made us a drink and did my washing-up for me. We were very close that afternoon and I was fully aware of the value of her friendship.

I had met Lesley some fifteen years ago. At that time I had had a smaller flat on the ground floor of the same block I was still living in. Lesley had a similar flat two floors above mine. Periodically the overflow of her toilet would disgorge itself of excess water which gushed out hitting the transom window of my lounge. I had rung on her doorbell several times, but as she was never in I put a light-hearted note through her door asking her to stop the flow. And so we met. She was teaching English and Drama in Borehamwood at the time. Some years later, being totally fed up with teaching, she got a job with Capital Radio on their Helpline. As time passed she decided that she did not want to be working at a pop radio station at the age of forty and took a job working to prevent drug abuse. From there she moved to the Health Authority as adviser for Sex, HIV and AIDS. Lesley liked to look stunning and she did not normally disappoint. We used to meet up more regularly in the first few years of our friendship, while she was still teaching. I remember sitting in her flat, which looked like a stage set, eating Camembert and grapes and watching *Soap* on the television. We still met up, though not so frequently, usually in my school holidays. The time we spent together was generally good.

So it wasn't until the following day that I went back to Surrey. I felt much better, but my legs were not quite right. I could walk and I could sit, but I couldn't stand still. The muscles just would not allow it. Washing, shaving and cleaning my teeth had to be interrupted every five seconds by a walk round the flat or a sit-down. Strange indeed.

My uncle David is a most remarkable man, fifty-five years old and quite the most energetic person I've ever met. He is in a league all by himself. I don't know him well. I remember him visiting us occasionally when I was little, but then he went to work in the States. He is a medical doctor and his specialism is infectious diseases which, of course, brings him into frequent contact with HIV and AIDS patients. He had come over on the different occasions when my father had been ill and spoken to the doctors. He had always impressed me.

Since I had left hospital I had spoken to him a couple of times on the phone, and he had endorsed all the treatments I had received, filling me in on one or two details which the clinic had probably thought beyond my comprehension. Inevitably the conversation when I arrived home revolved around my infection. He seemed to think it was a shame that I had not tested sooner, feeling that I could have been spared the pneumonia. He explained that the shuddering I had experienced on the Friday was known as the rigors, and was the body's way of dealing with its perception of a low temperature by contracting and expanding the muscles. The problem with my legs was as a result of dehydration following the vomiting. We talked and talked about my illness, about current affairs and about books (he is a tremendous reader. If it's been written he's read it and what is more remembers it, quite apart from his medical journals). Then we talked about Bill Clinton and his wife, Hillary. It was all getting too much for me, I was worn out and so, vacating my armchair, I went into the dining room to read. It was like having a whirlwind in the house.

The following morning at nine o'clock as I crept somewhat grumpily out of my room and headed towards the bathroom I met my mother coming out of the front bedroom. David, already up, had decided to teach himself Latin and she was fetching him some books to look at. That morning he told us all about the origins of Penicillin. As regards AIDS he felt a cure would be a fluke which might come today or not for a hundred years. In the meantime doctors were working towards providing cures for the various infections incurred by AIDS sufferers and extending their life spans in that way, so that AIDS, like arthritis, would become a chronic rather than a fatal condition. Before he left that afternoon he came up with a plan for me for the Septrin. He suggested that I should take just half a tablet to see if I had any tolerance of the drug at all. If I managed that I should take another half tablet and so on. He checked in a Journal he had brought with him the prophylactic dose of Septrin for pneumonia. If I could manage two tablets every day that was an equally good alternative to four tablets three days a week.

I wasn't expected back at the clinic now for a whole two weeks. The very next day I started again with the Septrin, just half a tablet after breakfast. I sat myself down in the lounge with my book and a bucket. After an hour I started feeling a bit strange in the head. After lunch I had another half tablet. No further reaction and after tea another half. In this way I managed to take one and a half tablets and I was all right. The next day I felt fine and took one whole tablet in the morning and again in the evening. This constituted the prophylactic dose and seemed like a minor triumph. I did start getting a bit spotty, but what the hell.

The following morning at a quarter to nine Professor Pasvol phoned. He had been trying to reach me in Stanmore. He told me they had found a little bug in my sputum which might account for my feeling so weary and would I come into the clinic? There was plenty of time for me to drive up that morning and see him in the afternoon, but I knew my mum was planning a pork casserole for our lunch and I didn't want to miss it so I made an appointment for the next morning.

Half way through the pork casserole the phone rang again. It was a Mrs Chater from the chest clinic ringing to ask about having the family checked. I said I didn't know what they were to be checked for as I hadn't seen Professor Pasvol yet. She wouldn't say, but I made an appointment to see her half an hour before I was due to see Professor Pasvol.

These two appointments were obviously the wrong way round, but Mrs Chater, who only works part-time, had to go out visiting later in the morning. I saw her at eleven o'clock, but she still wouldn't say what the matter was. She felt that my mother should be checked, because she was old, together with anyone else with whom I had frequent contact. I asked her about my colleagues at work and the children. Little children in particular sometimes come and stand very close to their teacher. She didn't consider it necessary. I gave her my mum's name and address and told her I would think about who else should be checked and let her know.

There was no sign of Professor Pasvol and I waited until nearly half past twelve. I went and had a word with Colette who apologised for the delay, and I was shown through to a rather harassed Dr Kapembwa. He explained that it was probably TB though that couldn't be finally confirmed until more tests were carried out. They had grown a culture from the sputum I had coughed up during my first few days in hospital. It takes between six and eight weeks to grow. He wanted me to start on the TB treatment straight away. He prescribed three drugs and a vitamin supplement. There was a fourth drug, but because it can cause problems with the vision I would need to have my eyes tested first. He would try to arrange for me to be seen by the ophthalmologist that afternoon. As it was nearly one o'clock I announced that I was going to the staff restaurant to have my lunch and that I would come back later. I chose Chinese beef on a bed of rice, I have never tasted anything like it and couldn't decide whether I liked it or not. I rather think not. The spotted dick and custard I had for pudding was superb. As I was leaving the dining room to take my coffee to the smoking area I bumped into Dr Davidson. He also knew about the TB. He said he thought it was just a very small colonisation. Again he had found the right words to cheer me up. As I drank my coffee I thought to myself. The pneumonia was history and I knew I had sufficient fight in me to give the TB a run for its money.

Back in the clinic I had to wait a while for the letter of introduction to Dr Bhide, the ophthalmologist, and then Colette accompanied me the one hundred yards down the corridor to the eye clinic. I waited until half past three. I felt dog-tired. I went up to the nurse on duty and said I was going back to the GUM clinic (Genito Urinary Medicine) for a cup of tea. Colette made me one and produced a splendid piece of cake to go with it. I was eventually seen at about four o'clock. I astounded the nurses by reading the bottom line of letters. With my lenses my distance vision is one hundred and twenty per cent. Then Dr Bhide performed various tests which included introducing some nasty drops into my eyes. He also tested me for colour blindness. I could only read the first two numbers and he confirmed that I had a defect in the red-green spectrum. He expressed surprise that I was able to make out traffic lights. The colour blindness was not a surprise to me. I had known about it since I was tested at junior school, but I had not realised how severe it was. I had to hang around for another half an hour before I could leave. The drops he had used anaesthetised the eyes and I wasn't to put my lenses back straight away. It was five o'clock when I left the hospital. I had been there six hours and I was ready to drop.

As resistant strains of TB have developed, the technique for treating it is to bombard it with different antibiotics. The cultures are all sent to one of the national TB centres (mine went to Dulwich), where they have the resources to regrow the cultures in order to find out the sensitivities of the strain. When this has been done, which takes another eight weeks, they know which drugs the strain responds to and can sometimes reduce the number of tablets.

I felt different as soon as I started the TB treatment. There were five tablets to be taken half an hour before breakfast and another five to be taken after breakfast and that was it. I was no longer weary in the morning, but around lunchtime I would start yawning and need a rest after lunch. It was only two days after starting treatment that I woke up one morning and decided to record what had happened to me since I first went to the doctor back in November. I have always enjoyed writing, but never felt that I had anything to say. Now I did. I have written furiously ever since. Every morning I have sat down to recall, as accurately as my memory allows, the events that have taken place; I have felt a great urgency to complete this task. It has not been easy as I have relived the whole episode and recalled my friendship with Howard and my father's death.

The day after I started writing I telephoned the theatre in Leatherhead, the Thorndike, to see if they still had seats for the Francis Durbridge thriller *Sweet Revenge*. They did and we went along that evening. Just as in the hospital some weeks before I felt self-conscious. The play was not very good and some of the acting not much better, but this was my first trip out and I was pleased to have gone.

Back in the clinic a couple of days later I saw Dr Kapembwa again. I went along with a long list of things to say and questions to ask. He decided because of my colour blindness not to prescribe the last TB drug. It is apparently the red-green spectrum which is critical and he feared permanent damage to my sight. I told him about the Septrin and how I had managed to take it. He looked at my face which was now quite bad with the rash and decided to stop the Septrin. I would have to use the nebuliser instead. I asked him whether there were any symptoms of the HIV that I should look out for that should cause me to ring the clinic. He mentioned difficulty swallowing, weakness in my limbs, a dry cough, night sweats, diarrhoea and a temperature. I asked him also whether there were any vaccinations I could have that might help ward off infection. This had been David's idea. As the immune system breaks down it finds it more difficult to produce antibodies, but he still thought it worth trying. Dr Kapembwa explained that the long-term vaccines were live vaccines which could cause problems with the HIV, and the dead vaccines were only short-term, such as one might have if going abroad. He did, however, think of two: Hepatitis B, which is genetically engineered, and Pneumococcus. He said he would look into it. Then I had my blood taken and had a go with the nebuliser. First of all I had to breathe in Ventolin for five minutes. This was to open up my lungs. Then Pentamidine. It took fifteen minutes and the machine looked just like a fan heater.

It was now nearly the end of January and when I weighed myself on the thirty-first I had reached ten stone. We bought a bottle of

Elderflower Champagne to celebrate. This is a local brew being made at Thorncroft Manor in Leatherhead.

There is a country house a couple of miles up the road from where we live in Fetcham. Polesden Lacey belonged to the Honourable Mrs Ronald Greville, well-known hostess, until her death in 1942. It is a very elegant building with marvellous gardens and extensive grounds. I remember going there as a child and the long walks we took. I used to like going to the little cemetery where Mrs Greville had buried her dogs. She herself was also buried in the grounds of the house. It amused me later when I learnt that she had buried her husband a mile or so away in Bookham churchyard. There is a little winter garden, and one sunny afternoon, of which we have had very few, my mum and I went to see the bulbs. The hundreds of little yellow winter aconites and lilac-coloured crocuses were at their best. It was a delight.

We were back in the theatre that week to see Joe Orton's play *Loot*. This was performed in the Casson Room and was superb. It was played to a much younger audience than the Francis Durbridge. I think many of them were drama students from the local college. At least, they all seemed to know one another and were wearing strange clothes.

I have had two part-time companions, Soldier and Tiger, next door's cats. Tiger is a dumpy little tabby who looks as if she is about to produce half a dozen kittens but never does. Soldier, who is Tiger's son, is long and black and couldn't be more different. Tiger is immensely affectionate and wants constantly to be stroked and cuddled. Soldier is far more wary. He always likes to have a yard or two between you and him. Then he gives you a look which says: "I would really rather like to be stroked too," but he is too proud. They sit huddled together in our front porch looking like two tea cosies and stretch and bask in the sun if it is a nice day.

My visits to the clinic have become less frequent. I still have to go once a month to have my blood checked and to use the nebuliser. I am asked the usual questions each time. Any diarrhoea, rashes, fevers? Any trouble swallowing? I have had one or two little problems but nothing serious. Since I started the TB treatment my eyes have been dry. The folliculitis causes me to itch at night and I wake very early. I will be continuing with the AZT for the rest of my days or until a better drug supersedes it. The TB treatment will take nine months. What saddens me is the fact that when I am cured of the TB I will still not be well as the underlying problem remains. Curiously the AZT, which is an anti-viral treatment, seems to have cured a large, nasty verruca on my foot which I have had for years. I have noticed that my nails have started growing again and my hair, which had become quite sparse, is getting thicker.

I have continued to eat well and hope that my weight may reach eleven stone. I feel sure that this will afford some measure of protection for me. I have a little booklet entitled *Eating for HIV*. It is essential to eat a lot of protein: meat, fish, eggs, cheese, twice a day. Forget low-fat spreads; milk, butter and cream are what you need. Essentially though I have continued to eat a well-balanced diet which I have supplemented each afternoon with a glass of Nestlé's Build Up, which contains essential minerals and vitamins.

Part Three

It is the 1st March, St David's Day, and it is perhaps time to stop for a moment and to reflect. The clinic has sorted out my medication though we are still waiting to hear back from the national TB centre. It will take about another month before we have the sensitivities. I weighed myself last night - ten and a half stone. I still have the shadow on my lung, but most of the time I now feel in good health (though I won't admit it). This is in itself confusing when the virus which has enabled the pneumonia, TB and thrush to get a hold is still working away inside me. I have decided that I don't like the virus very much, but it is powerful and I respect it. However, it must not be allowed to become autonomous and we must learn somehow to live together in my body. I cannot truthfully say that it is welcome, but if it treats me gently I think we can get along. If not we are both the losers.

Now that I have realised that I am not immediately dying (which I certainly thought until I saw Dr Davidson at the beginning of January) my attitude towards HIV and AIDS has changed somewhat. Initially I had felt I did not want to know too much (I suppose because I was frightened) and I had frequently interrupted the doctors and Karen saying: "I don't want to know". I feel now I would like to inform myself a little about the virus and its mechanisms. I haven't got very far with this because as soon as I start reading about it I am immediately confronted with the different and horrific illnesses and problems it can cause. I am too frightened then to carry on reading. I am scared most by the skin tumours. In fact I have even blotted the name of these from my mind. I do not want to see my body mutilated by these unsightly marks. If I do get them I will find it difficult to go on fighting. One of the books on AIDS shows on its front cover a photograph of a man's back which is covered with these tumours. It looks obscene. I have realised that the symptoms that I have had, the dermatitis, thrush, pneumonia and TB mean that I have AIDS or at least ARC (AIDS Related Complex). I find this difficult to accept and prefer to think of myself as just HIV positive. The word AIDS for me is synonymous with hopelessness and death and so I will be remaining just HIV positive.

The shock horror of learning that I was positive has now passed and I am managing to get on with my life. Probably the writing has helped me in this. It is something new and important in my life. I do not constantly think about HIV and AIDS anymore. When I am reading or watching TV I have no trouble concentrating on my book or the programme. The novelty has, I suppose, worn off. There are moments, however, when I feel down, I am finished, that I have reached the end. I feel sometimes resigned to my death. I even think that if I am going to die then the sooner the better. These moments are infrequent and I am ashamed of them, particularly when I think of the tremendous efforts the doctors are making in order to keep me fit and well, but I must own up to them. They are real. Mostly I suppose I am frightened of the illnesses I have inadvertently read about and imagine I will have them all at once, and I still need to talk a great deal about the infection.

Life has become very precious, and I am aware of each extra day that I have been granted. I don't want to miss anything. When I came home from the hospital the snowdrops were already in bloom and I have watched the crocuses and them, and now the daffodils, come out. I have watched the trees come into blossom and I have watched the birds in the garden. We have had two woodpeckers: the green and the greater spotted and a jay. I have seen the foxes and all the neighbouring cats going about their business. I have observed them all with new eyes, for I realise I may never see them again, and I don't want anything to escape me.

I am treating this year as my last though I hope that it won't be. And so how does one spend one's last year? What are the things that I still want to do? I have no great desire to travel. Since I was young and used to plan our holidays with my father I have never again really enjoyed holidays. What I want is to watch the changes of the seasons, the flowers and the trees flourish in all their splendour and then die back and conserve their energy in order then next year to flourish anew. I want to watch the animals and the birds and the insects, all the living things. If I go away then I want to go somewhere where I can swim in the sea; where I can go snorkelling and see the brightly coloured fish in their underwater world. If I come back in another incarnation I should quite like to be a fish and swim around in a shoal of friends. I want to feel in harmony with the world I shall be leaving.

What have I learnt in the last three months? That I love life. That I love nature. That I love the people around me. I have learnt also to let them love me and do things for me. My mother has of course provided everything for me just as when I was a child, but I think also of the toast and honey that Mike made me, the washing-up Lesley did for me. I am borne along by the warmth and kindness of all these people and the diligence of my doctors.

"I am never going back." I had said this so many times. Back in November to Karen and to Dr Kapembwa. Innumerable times since to various people. In fact, I had said it so many times that I had begun to doubt that I meant it. During the last three months, despite my illness, I had felt happier than I had in many years. I hated my job.

When I was at university I spent the third year of my course as a Languages Assistant in Bonn. I had a marvellous time. It was a grammar school with both boarders and day pupils. It was absolutely right for me, I fitted in perfectly. I took classes for my German colleagues who were grateful to be relieved of some of their burden. My lessons were good, the children interested. I was only twenty-one, but I had no discipline problems at all. I even taught one class of Latin for a while when their teacher was sick. I joined in fully with the life of the boarding school going out with groups of children at weekends. I loved it and so I decided to go into teaching.

I did my teaching practice in Chigwell and then joined my present school some seventeen years ago. This was a different cup of tea entirely. I had never seen behaviour like this before; it was like working in a penitentiary. There were some good classes and some very nice children, but, apart from the first years, who were fun to be with and who tried quite hard, life was a battle from start to finish. There were very disruptive children in nearly all classes who constantly drew attention to themselves, spoiled the lessons for the others and prevented them from getting on. I felt very sorry for the children who did want to learn. However, there was one group I taught, year ten German, who would come into the classroom and get their books out and wait for me to start my lesson. The lessons were conducted in almost total silence as they sat and applied themselves to the work in hand. I mention this solely as it was so unusual, so exceptional and wonderful that it quite disarmed me at the time. I even convinced myself that they didn't like me, but that was very far from the truth. They were just keen to get on and enjoyed their German.

I remember having classes with children who wouldn't even come into the room. In such cases, when no one was prepared to listen, the best thing to do was to go in and write some work on the board in the hope that some people would make a start, and then go round and bully, persuade and cajole others to get their books out and have a go. The language that some of them used was frightful. Some wandered round the room like primary school children. You have no idea how exhausting just thirty-five minutes can be in a classroom with thirty children of moderate to low ability who are always bored, foulmouthed and sometimes violent in class. I wonder sometimes whether in all those years I ever taught anyone anything. I certainly never learned the meaning of job satisfaction.

No wonder I didn't want to go back, but I fretted constantly about it, and most nights in my dreams I was back there battling with a headmaster who, I was convinced, didn't like me. My mortgage was very small and I had a lot of money saved, but it really wasn't enough to give up work entirely if I was going to last more than a couple of years. I remembered my Uncle David's warning: "How will you look in six years' time if you've given up your job and you're still going strong?" Nor did I really want just to sit around waiting to die. Had the job not been so exhausting and so ghastly I would have been quite keen to go back. I had said to myself initially, before the TB was discovered, that I would go back at the beginning of March. Then I decided that I would try to stop fretting about it and definitely not return until the beginning of the Summer Term. But that is only six weeks away now and I am thinking that perhaps I should wait until the beginning of the new 'academic' year in September. That would allow me time to build myself up and create a margin of health to cushion me when I do go back. I would also have a few months to enjoy myself while I am still in good health.

There were perhaps other options that I should look into. There was the possibility of early retirement or to return part-time. It was still too early to make a decision. I did not yet know how good I was going to feel or how tired I would get, but it did not stop my fretting. Should I perhaps apply to Hertfordshire County Council for an administrative post instead, backed up by a letter from Dr Kapembwa stating that he didn't want me to return to teaching for health reasons? I really didn't know what to do.

Next August we will have been living in this house for forty years. We moved in on my second birthday. When I was five I went to the Primary School at the bottom of the road. It was a strange-looking building, a bit like a chapel. It was opposite the pub. We were all very small, but Miss Chipping, the reception class teacher, was only a couple of inches taller than us. On Sundays I also used to go there in the morning for Sunday School. This was my first connection with the Church, and I remember sitting there listening to the wonderful stories from the Bible and then singing *All things bright and beautiful* while someone thumped out the tune on the piano. When I was older I became a choir boy. We used to practise every Thursday evening with Mr Clark and sing in church at the eleven o'clock service on Sunday. When I was fourteen I was confirmed. I remember this particularly well as it was the day of the Aberfan disaster and was nearly postponed. I continued going to church regularly until I left home when I was seventeen, I would still quite like to go, but I do not really feel part of a community either in Stanmore or in Fetcham.

The old vicar, Mr Maby, had passed away and been succeeded by the Reverend Baker whom I have arranged to see this afternoon. I rang up yesterday morning and I have an appointment at two-thirty. I told my mother about this appointment. I think it has quite upset her. She told me that I must be positive. Perhaps it's unnecessary. I certainly hope it's premature, but I would hate to be 'put away' by someone who didn't even know me. It also seems to me a courtesy to him as I wish to be buried in his patch.

This morning I woke up wishing I hadn't made the appointment. It feels all wrong, I feel superstitiously that it will hasten my death. I should have spoken instead to Dick. He was Head of Science until he retired a couple of years ago. He had taken Holy Orders and was now working in a parish in Bedfordshire. He was someone who knew me and liked me. I think I would feel more comfortable with him.

Anyway I'm stuck with this appointment now, I can't very well ring up and say that I've decided not to die. What am I going to say? I shall probably start by apologising, saying that my visit is perhaps unnecessary, I shall tell him that I've been ill, still am, that I am HIV positive, that I hope I'll have a few years yet, but I feel that my condition is unpredictable. I shall tell him about my connection with St Mary's and ask him about the cremation. I want to choose some music and have a poem read out. Perhaps I'll be able to get away in half an hour. I just want him to have met me. Oh dear, I wish I hadn't arranged this.

I'm really glad I went. I feel I have staked my claim or perhaps restaked it here in Fetcham, at church, in the cemetery. I know that if I want to go to church here I will be welcome. I explained to Mr Baker about my illnesses and the HIV, expressed my hope and intention of carrying on for a few years yet, but explained that I wanted him to know who I was so that, at a later date, he didn't feel he had a stranger in the churchyard. He told me that he was sixty-five and would perhaps be retiring in a couple of years. He told me about his career and I told him about my teaching. He was originally a professional musician; his instrument was the piano. He started out at St Albans Cathedral as Music Master and then moved to Friern Barnet to complete his education, as he put it. Then he had a parish at Tattenham Corner for twelve years before coming to Fetcham where he had been for nine and a half years. I asked him about the cremation, saying that I wanted some music to be played and a poem read out. He thought this a very good idea. He said that it made his job easier if someone had expressed their wishes in this way. He urged me to write down what I wanted and make sure people knew where it was. He reminded me that the only certainty in life is death. I kept it fairly light-hearted, but he got my message and I was away in half an hour. I went to see the tablet where my father's ashes are interred. I placed my hand on the stone and told him about the HIV; I'm sure he forgave me. Then I went to see Mr Maby's stone. I am so glad I went.

When my time comes I will take my turn, graciously I hope, and those whom I loved so much and whose parting caused me so many tears will be there to welcome me. My grandmother, we called her Ninny, will be there with her brother Non, who died in the first war, but who was always in her thoughts. They'll be watching the television together (probably *University Challenge*) with a box of Black Magic chocolates in my grandmother's lap. My father will be there too. Eleanor says he will be talking to Shakespeare, Bill and Will together. Perhaps too he will have met for the first time his own father who was reported missing presumed killed on the very day my father was born, again in the First World War. And what a reunion Howard and I will have. He is probably talking to God himself right now confusing even Him with one of his infinitely long stories. God will be glad when I arrive so that He can go about His business again.

Others will follow me, my mum, my sister, friends, relatives, colleagues, lovers. And we will have a party like there never was. But until then I must get on with my life.

At the beginning of February I had a dream. I dreamed that I was standing at a bar buying a round of drinks. Whatever I asked for, the barman got the order wrong. It was taking ages. Then I was buying crisps and things. Again he got it wrong. The same thing happened when I came to pay. Eventually I returned to my table with the drinks. There were the four of us. Clive and I were together and Stuart and someone else. I lent forward to Clive and whispered in his ear: "HIV," and then in his other ear I whispered: "AIDS."

I knew I must ring him and tell him about my infection. I put it off for a couple of weeks, but the dream was haunting me and eventually I rang. He was shocked, but remained quite calm.. I told him I would like to see him. I told him I would rather see him alone if that were possible. He took the following Friday off work and came up in the afternoon. It was marvellous to see him and not only because he had brought a superb raspberry torte with him. I told him what had been happening. I told him that I was sorry that things hadn't worked out between him and me, said that I knew it had been partly my fault. We chatted for a couple of hours. I showed him my photographs of Madeira where I had been last Summer. It was fun, it always is fun when Clive and I are together. I could not hold back my tears as he was leaving.

Julian said a strange thing to me when I came out of hospital. I didn't mention it at the time because I did not realise the significance of what he was saying. It was at the beginning of January when I returned to Stanmore for my first clinic appointment. He knew I was coming back and when he rang on the Wednesday I said: "How about Friday evening?" "Well, I don't know. Things have changed while you were away." I shrugged it off at the time. He did in fact come round and has continued to come on Friday evening when I have been in Stanmore. Then, about the middle of February, he announced that he had been to France for the day. It seemed strange to me because I had had lunch with him only a couple of days before and he hadn't mentioned it. I asked him who he had gone with. He was cagey. "A chap I met in a pub." I didn't pursue my interrogation, Julian and I are not lovers, but I was upset. I have no claim on him except perhaps that of friendship. I think I was upset by his secrecy and I felt I was being replaced before I was even in the box.

There is one other person, whom I have not mentioned so far, who has, as yet, no idea of my illness. I met him about ten years ago within days of meeting Julian. He was twelve years older than me. I think it is fair to say he fell in love with me. He would ring me up every day, some days several times. I liked him. It was difficult to meet up. He would come to my flat when I was on holiday and spend the day with me. He usually brought champagne. On other occasions we would meet in Bushy Park and go and have lunch or a drink. One of his hobbies was painting. He did two paintings for me, one of St Mary's and one of my old primary school. I had to buy these at the local exhibition in order not to arouse suspicion. I grew accustomed to him and his phone calls. I grew to depend on them and I grew to love him. Then, one Easter holiday, after I had known him for a couple of years, I went away to Germany for ten days. During that time he found someone else. His phone calls became less frequent and I could tell he did not feel comfortable speaking to me. When we met up in the summer he could not look me in the eye. In October he came up to Bedfordshire on a course and we arranged to meet. We spent what I thought was a good evening together and I returned to the flat. I went to bed and was asleep when the phone rang. He said he was having a breakdown and couldn't see me anymore. I was very upset, but Howard was very supportive of me. When he was back in the office I rang him again. He made an excuse, but didn't ring back. I sent him a Christmas card and received one in return. Eventually, through my efforts I suppose, we resumed telephone contact. I would hear from him every couple of months or so. Very occasionally we met for a drink. I felt he was deceiving himself about how he felt towards me. We still talk once in a while. I don't feel the same way about him any more. I don't look forward to his calls, but I enjoy them when they come. The last time we spoke was October. I am sure he will have tried ringing me since, but I haven't been in Stanmore very much. I can't ring him at home and last October he took early retirement and so there is no work number now. I think I want him to know that I'm not well, I would like to feel close to him again as we were eight or ten years ago. I will wait for him to call, unless I get ill again, and then I'll call him.

Part Four

My reflections were interrupted at ten past six on Friday, 5th March by a telephone call from Dr Kapembwa. He said he felt my latest X-ray was lagging behind. What he meant was that he thought my pneumonia had returned. He wanted me to come into hospital the following week to have a biopsy of the shadow on my lung. He didn't know what it was and feared it might be triggering the pneumonia. He explained briefly the procedure: a needle through my back into the lung. Would I feel anything? Just the sting of the local anaesthetic. He hoped it wouldn't spoil my weekend.

I went into the lounge, turned off *The Six o'clock News*, looked at my mum and burst into tears. It was the shock. I thought I had been doing so well. Later on I phoned my sister to tell her, but, realising she was more upset than me, I desisted. She had been to the doctor about a little lump on her eyelid, a bit like a pea. He had told her it was a cyst and that she would have to have it removed surgically, either under a local anaesthetic or, because she is a very nervous person, a general. My concern for her and her great anxiety enabled me to put my problems in perspective. After all I was only going in for tests and I was going back to a ward where I had felt quite comfortable and happy.

I only told a handful of people, Julian, Lesley, Mike and Mike, Clive. I told them I didn't want visitors. I thought that I would be busy the whole time with the tests and I wanted to be able to focus my attention on these without interruption. I said I would ring if I wanted them to visit.

I got my bag ready, packing my essentials, the radio, *The Radio Times*, and my cigarettes, and set out on Monday morning for the hospital. It was a lovely sunny day, the first day of spring. I sat in the hospital car park in the sun smoking a cigarette and listening to a tape. I had decided to take the car this time because I did not intend staying long. If it got damaged or stolen, so be it, it was insured. Clarke Ward in the Lister Unit had been closed. In fact it had been closed the afternoon I was discharged two days before Christmas. It wasn't to reopen until April, the beginning of the new financial year. I was heading for Byrd Ward which was a floor lower, but in all other respects identical. The sun was streaming through the glass into the room when I arrived and it was already hot in there. The first person I met was Chris. She is middle-aged, husband in the RAF and has decided she wants to go into nursing so she is training at Northwick Park. She gave me a hug. All my other friends were there too: Kim, Tanya, Mairead, Juanita, Louise and two young men, Mark and Eamon. I couldn't settle down that morning. I had an apple and unpacked my things and then wandered along to the staff restaurant for a coffee. It was only now on my return in good health that I realised how ill and how weak I had been in December. I hadn't been aware of it at the time. Fortunately things are hidden from us.

I had woken very early that morning and so in the afternoon I was quite content to lie on the bed and listen to the play, a murder mystery. I had about three interruptions. Tanya came in to fill in a form and then Dr Witty, the ward doctor, brought the form of consent for the biopsy and told me what could go wrong. The lung could puncture, it could collapse. I'd rather he hadn't told me, but he is obliged to. Professor Pasvol came and examined me. It was very difficult to follow the play because I kept having to switch it off and I never did find out who the murderer was. In the evening I saw Dr Kapembwa. He works at St Mary's hospital on Tuesdays and his clinic does not finish until four o'clock. As he wanted to be present during my biopsy he had arranged for it to take place at five o'clock the following day so that he would be able to get back to Northwick Park.

I didn't relish the idea of a needle passing through my back into my lung and I was very anxious. In fact my pulse was raised the next morning. How was I going to spend the day waiting until five o'clock with nothing to do? At a quarter to nine Hans, a German student who was spending a term at Northwick Park, came into my room and asked if I minded him asking me questions. He was a pleasant chap and was with me for at least three quarters of an hour. He ran through the whole of my medical history with me and I taught him how to say pneumonia.

When he'd gone, I went for a wander round the ward to stretch my legs. The tea lady, who recognised me from December, told me I was getting fat. I was ever so pleased. Then I saw Jenny Bagnell, the lay-preacher, coming into the ward. We had had a long chat together in December. She came into my room and I told her how I had been getting on. We talked for about an hour. I had watched a programme on the television the night before, *A Secret World of Sex*. It was about syphilis. It had made me think. Sixty thousand people in Britain died each year from syphilis in the 1920s, and the mass infection of the troops even threatened to undermine the Allied war effort until the discovery of Penicillin in 1943. It made me realise that what I had done wasn't really so bad. Thousands of other people had died from their enjoyment of sex who had not even had AIDS. Up till then my attitude had been that my infection was my own fault and that I must take the punishment. I discussed this with her and came to understand how judgmental I had been. Having sex wasn't bad even if, as in my case, it had led to HIV infection. This was an important revelation for me.

I went along to the restaurant to have my coffee and came back as lunch was being served. I was just tucking in when I had another visitor, Cathy Ryan, the social worker. She stayed with me while I ate my lunch and I discussed my job situation with her. She was very helpful and gave me a lot of practical advice. She suggested that I should ring the personnel department at County Hall to ask about early retirement or the possibility of a less rigorous job. She suggested that I should get in touch with the Terrence Higgins Trust. She thought I should have a chat with Dr Kapembwa to try to find out what my state of health was likely to be. Those were all sound practical ideas.

I had just watched *Neighbours'*, lunchtime showing, when I had yet another visitor. I had told everyone how anxious I was and I started thinking that all these visitors were just a ploy to keep my mind off the afternoon's procedure. Adrian, like Hans, was a student. He went through my medical history and he was just examining me when Dr Witty appeared. He explained to me what the problem was with my X-ray. White fluffy stuff had appeared at the bottom of my lung. He wanted me to have a bronchoscopy the next morning and had brought the form for my consent. I wasn't keen on the idea of having another procedure the following day, but I knew that bronchoscopies were Mondays and Wednesdays so I signed my agreement.

I was given a couple of pills and warned not to attempt to move from my bed. The porter took me down to the CT room at about a quarter to four. I stretched out on my stomach with my hands in front grasping what looked like a miniature set of handlebars and Dr Mitchell gave me a scan. 'Breathe in, hold your breath, relax,' It was the same recorded voice that I remembered from December. I did my best, but I was fighting against the pills and kept nodding off. Then came the biopsy. I wasn't to move a whisker. They kept me waiting as they worked out precisely where the needle was to go on. My shoulders and chest were aching like mad from my unnatural extension. Eventually I felt the prick of the needle with the local anaesthetic. They went in three times, with a thump negotiating a rib on the way in. The second time when they got inside my lung it hurt. It hurt a lot. If it hadn't been for those pills I would have got up and said: "Enough's enough," and marched out, but they were making me dopey. Afterwards I was taken along to be X-rayed and brought back to the ward, feeling a bit tender inside. It had not been a pleasant experience, but all was well and the pulse oximeter showed that my oxygen saturation was one hundred per cent. I decided that I wouldn't let them do this again.

That night before the bronchoscopy, I decided to have a couple of sleeping pills in the hope that I wouldn't wake too early the next morning. This worked, but I also dreamed. I dreamed about David. It was not a nice dream. We were on a boat and he was ignoring me.

No breakfast, not even a cup of tea, but I did sneak a quick fag. How long would I have to wait? I hadn't even cleaned my teeth when Eamon came to give me my pre-med at a quarter to nine. Within minutes the porter was there to wheel my bed down. The bronchoscopy room, which on the previous two occasions had been sunk in darkness apart from a Sony monitor next to the bed, was brightly lit this time with fluorescent lights. Hanging on the wall behind the monitor like dog leads were different-sized tubes. Rob Wilkinson had gone to the Sudan; someone told me he had gone there to sort out a strange chest infection. Dr Millidge, the consultant, was to do the honours today. When he came in I was sitting up in bed. I drew his attention to the fact that I had had a biopsy the day before hoping that he would go into a different part of my lung. He said to one of the nurses that the pre-med didn't seem to have had much effect on me and he gave me a shot in the arm. We were ready to go. I was attached to the pulse oximeter to measure my oxygen saturation. I snorted up as much gel as I could and someone remarked that I had obviously done this before. The thing in my nose, which hadn't bothered me before, was very uncomfortable and so he decided to go in through the other nostril. I seem to have been much more aware of what was going on this time. The bright lights didn't help. I watched him the whole time, his steady hand, and listened to what he was saying. I was aware of the probe in my lung and could feel the picking sensation inside when he did the biopsy. It was an uncomfortable and unpleasant experience. At one point the nurse had to give me oxygen. When he finished I sat up on the side of the bed swinging my legs. The nurses were worried I might fall off. I waited there talking to them for quite a while before the porter came to take me back to my room. "Where's my cup of tea?" I asked Eamon straight away, but I wasn't allowed a drink for a couple of hours until the anaesthetising gel had worn off.

I dozed in bed until a quarter past twelve. Eamon brought me a beaker of water. I sat up and took a little sip, just enough to disperse in my mouth. It tasted better than wine. I took a few more sips. Then the pain in my chest started. It was sudden and unexpected and I was flustered. Eamon got me some pain killers and fetched Dr Witty. By this time I was sweating heavily from the pain and my anxiety. The pain killers took a couple of hours to take effect. I was glad when they did. Later that afternoon I was taken for an X-ray. The lung had punctured during the biopsy and I had a small Pneumothorax. This is when air escapes from the lung into the cavity surrounding it. The air is then gradually reabsorbed by the lung though this can take several days. In severe cases a drainage tube has to be inserted into the lung though this can apparently cause problems in AIDS patients.

That evening I was sitting in my room, relieved that the two procedures were over and feeling a bit sorry for myself when Clive walked in. I burst into tears. There was no one in the world that I would have rather seen. I told him about the biopsies and then we sat eating the chocolates he had brought and talking. I feel comfortable with Clive and there is still a great deal of affection between us. That night, after more pain killers, I decided that the next time I needed a bronchoscopy I would go to the Sudan. Dr Wilkinson had been gentler.

The Thursday I had a leisurely day, listening to the radio and going for cups of coffee. There was a programme about Diana Gould, the Cirencester housewife, who had rattled Mrs Thatcher back in 1983 over the sinking of the Belgrano. There was another about Baroness Stocks . While I was wandering round the ward I met the sister of the lady in the next room. She had been on holiday in Tenerife and had suddenly gone blind. I learned later from Dr Davidson that she had a bacterial infection, but that the damage to her eyes was so great that she wouldn't recover her sight. I hadn't met her, but I felt very sorry for her. I thought to myself that I would perhaps rather be HIV positive than lose my sight, but I wasn't sure. Later in the afternoon I resolved to walk round outside to the front of the hospital. It was still lovely and sunny, but I only got a couple of hundred yards before the pain in my chest returned and I had to make my way gingerly back to the ward and ask for more pain killers.

On Friday, Dr Heyderman, the chief registrar, came to see me. I could go home that evening or Saturday morning. That morning I saw the lady from the next room. She was a blonde lady and was walking back into the ward escorted by Eamon. She was holding a daffodil which someone had given her. How dreadful that she couldn't see it, but only feel it and smell it. In the afternoon Dr Heyderman reappeared with a group of about six finals students which included Adrian and Hans. Would I mind if they practised on me? Not at all. It was always nice to be the centre of attention. He told them to auscultate, which meant listen to my chest. I tried to organise them into a competition. Whoever could tell me what was wrong with my chest could have a coffee cream. I had treated myself to a box of Black Magic chocolates and had eaten them all apart from two coffee creams which I don't like. Hans and Adrian already knew, but no one else would hazard a guess. I offered them the coffee creams anyway, but no one appeared to like them. Perhaps I should write to Rowntree. I hung around all day waiting for the results from the tests they had done. They were looking for three things: pneumonia, a fungal infection and TB. All the tests were negative. They would now have to go for culture. I was disappointed. I could see the problem on the X-ray myself and was hoping that they would have found out what it was and be able to treat it. At least the pneumonia wasn't back.

I had my tea and then set off home at about seven o'clock. I was hoping that Lesley would be in to help me carry my bags up to the flat. She wasn't. I took them up one by one, but I was panting by the time I reached the flat. I felt miserable, coming home with my Pneumothorax and there was no one there and I had had no results. In addition it had been quite fun in hospital. I hadn't been ill and had enjoyed the company of all the nurses. Eamon and Mark had looked after me, most of the time. They were marvellous. My meals had been cooked for me and I had been able to do as I pleased. I hoped that Julian might ring and come round. He didn't, but I did hear from Mike and Mike and Clive.

I was up early the next day and feeling more positive. I had resolved that I was not going to become a permanent invalid or else there seemed no point to the time I had left. After lunch I went for a little walk. I walked at a snail's pace for about half a mile. My chest was still quite tender. I sat on a bench in the sun. During my week in hospital the season had changed. Winter had become Spring. Everywhere there were hundreds of celandines showing their bright little faces. There were insects, midges, bees and there was the rustling of mice in the undergrowth. It was good to be alive.

Sunday was a nice day too. I went round to see Peter in the afternoon. He had had a dreadful car crash two days after Christmas and was lucky to be alive. The shock of the impact had also caused his prostate to pack up. Anyway he was back now, out of plaster and peeing like a cart-horse. We went for a walk with his dog. Elsa is a cross between a black Labrador and a collie, and has boundless energy. Peter limped along and I crept along beside him. We walked about a mile and then went back to his house and swapped hospital tales like two old men.

When I left the hospital I had been given strict instructions that if I had any problems breathing or any shortness of breath at all I was immediately to come back to the hospital. This was the reason I had stayed in Stanmore rather than going down to stay with my mum. She had decided to come and visit me on the Monday and I was looking forward to seeing her again. As usual I woke very early. I don't know whether it was the prospect of entertaining her for the day and cooking lunch that seemed more than I could cope with, but I felt terribly miserable and depressed. When she arrived I felt I had nothing to say and didn't cheer up until just before lunch. I turned to her and said: "I feel like I'm fighting a fight which is already lost." Having managed to articulate this I began to pick up a bit. We had a nice walk in the sunshine and I took her back to the station.

I still felt quite low, just wished I could have one day off, just one day when I did not have to carry the burden of knowing I was HIV positive. I was seeing Eva at five o'clock. She suggested that my depression was perhaps because of all the internal physical intrusion I had suffered the week before. That evening I sat down and wrote a letter to Dr Kapembwa. I wanted him to do something to tackle the HIV. I wanted him to be bold, to be innovative in my treatment, not to give in to it.

18th March, 1993

Dear Dr Kapembwa

One day one person will be cured of HIV. It maybe next week, it maybe in one hundred years, but it will happen. And when it is cured thirteen million more can also be cured.

Since I first came to your clinic I have received outstanding treatment and care. You have addressed the pneumonia and TB and put me on AZT. With luck I'll last a few years. You have already saved my life by curing the pneumonia.

From your involvement with HIV over the years and your research I am certain that you have ideas or even hunches which you would like to put into practice. I am resilient and I want to urge you to be bold, to be aggressive in my treatment. I want to give you the opportunity to try out these ideas, these hunches in order to find out more about HIV.

There is no reason on earth why the first person to be cured, and cured one day they will be, should not be at Northwick Park and I want you to be assured of my full cooperation in any treatments and my keen participation in any experiments you may like to carry out.

You can ignore this letter, but I needed to write it so that you are aware of the full extent of my commitment and also my gratitude, I am offering the greatest contribution I can possibly make - myself - and I hope you will hear what I am saying, take me at my word and use this opportunity I am giving you.

You may like to draw this letter to the attention of Professor Pasvol and Dr Davidson so that they are also aware of how I feel.

Yours sincerely

The next morning I reread the letter. Could I give it to him? I wasn't sure how he would react and I didn't want to antagonise him. I was still depressed. Then I got it into my head to find out how I had got the infection in the first place. There were only two people I thought I could have got it from. I looked up Phil's telephone number and then I checked my database for John's. It wasn't there so I checked the backup files. Still no luck. I phoned directory enquiries. No success. I rang Phil's number. If he were sick he might be at home. I got the answering machine. I heard his voice again and heard his silly message. I hung up. I realised that I didn't want to have anything more to do with him. He had already caused sufficient chaos in my life. I couldn't risk it again. One stupid idea was followed by another. I had been given the hospital discharge letter for my doctor. It was sealed. I opened it. It was after all about me. I recognised Dr Witty's writing. Main diagnosis: AIDS. I could have coped if he had written HIV or Retroviral Infection but I did not want to see this, a written confirmation that I was dying. Underneath, in his very scrappy writing, he had listed the procedures I had had and mentioned the Pneumothorax. By this time my mood was absolutely black.

Those were the worst two days I have had so far. I don't really know why, nor why my spirits then picked up. Wednesday morning I drove into Watford to get some computer stationery and had an argument with the man in the shop. I delivered the discharge letter to my doctor. I wanted it out of my flat. In the afternoon I had my hair cut and put the car through the car wash. Then I started work on the roof garden. The troughs and tubs were all still piled up in one corner from the previous November when Kevin had come to resurface it. It was a beautiful, sunny afternoon. I put the tubs and troughs back to their proper places. They were heavy, but I managed. I weeded round the roses and fertilised the soil. I was out there for a couple of hours working just in my shirt sleeves. I felt so much better.

The next morning I was at the garden centre by half past nine. I have always wanted to have a blue rose. I bought one once. It was five years ago, but then my father got ill and I didn't get round to putting it in. When my father died I discovered that the rose was also dead. Anyway there they were. Blue Moon. I chose a good strong plant and I also bought a lupin. I drove back and planted the rose. I hope that I will see it bloom.

That evening Julian came round. We had just started on the wine when the phone rang. It was David. I told him to sit down and then I told him I had AIDS. I could hear how shocked he was. He kept saying: "Oh shit," and I kept talking so he wouldn't have to say anything. I told him I had wanted to tell him and had been waiting for him to ring. I told him how I had been in hospital with the pneumonia. I told him about the TB and I told him about the biopsies. I also said very firmly that I wasn't finished yet. He was the only person I had told who had reacted in front of me. I cannot tell what my mother and my sister really felt or my friends and colleagues. They kept their feelings close to their chests. I felt elated that he had rung, but I couldn't get off to sleep that night.

The sun was still shining when I drove down to my mother the next morning. I was in the best of spirits. Whizzing round the M25 I thought to myself: 'I'm lucky', I know that I am going to die, not immediately, but in the next few years. I have the opportunity to use the time I have left to the very best of my ability, to enjoy what the world has to offer and to be conscious of that enjoyment, to love and appreciate the people around me, to do my writing. For most people when they realise they are dying it is already too late. Either they die suddenly or they are too ill to do the things I can still do. For me also there is a chance of a last minute reprieve, a fluke cure, a *deus ex machina*, though I would be a fool to count on it.

At home the flowers in the garden were marvellous. The daffs were still going strong and the tulips and the hyacinths had come out - what a fragrance. The trittoleia (my father's favourites) were in bloom and so were the anemones and the tiny scillas and chionodoxa (my favourites). We have had over a week of nearly uninterrupted sunshine and that in the middle of March. We returned to Polesden Lacey for a wander round. I can hardly wait to see the rose gardens when they come into bloom later in the year.

What then were the results of the tests that I had during my week in hospital? Dr Kapembwa was off on leave for a couple of weeks so my first appointment was with the Professor. They had at last heard back from the national TB centre. I had an atypical mycobacterial infection. It was not tuberculosis, but mycobacterium Xenopi. It was described to me as a quirky, environmental bug which crops up occasionally and which one might pick up from stagnant water. To most people it is harmless, but being immuno-suppressed I had succumbed to it. I hadn't caught it off anyone and I couldn't pass it on; I resolved to be more particular about throwing out the washing up water when I had finished with it. Howard used to tease me about this and I used to tell him that it had to last all week. They didn't have the sensitivities yet. That would take longer as sub-cultures now had to be grown. Like tuberculosis it is intracellular growing in the heart of the cells and taking equally long to cure. Some mycobacteria are exquisitely sensitive, others are more resistant, but they are all treatable.

It was still too soon for the results of the biopsy and the bronchoscopy, but the Professor did tell me what my CD4 count was. The CD4 or 'helper' cells are central to the immune system and this count shows how far the infection has progressed. In normal, healthy people the count is between six hundred and a thousand. In HIV patients when it drops to two hundred they start giving AZT and also begin the prophylaxis for pneumonia. My count in February had been eighty. This didn't sound very good, but it had risen from December when, apparently, it had only been forty. I felt quite pleased. More important for me was the fact that the Professor had said he thought I looked quite sparkling. You have no idea how important little comments like this have been and how much they have boosted me, I sparkled off home feeling wonderful.

The following Thursday I saw Dr Davidson. He now had the results from my tests. The bronchoscopy had revealed nothing except that I appeared to be clear of the pneumonia. The biopsy showed a blood clot with certain foreign cells in it. It was described to me as a benign tumour, like a polyp. I was again told that it was nothing to worry about, but that they would keep an eye on it. It wasn't HIV-related. I didn't believe this last comment. To my mind everything about me is now HIV-related. If my toes dropped off I would blame the HIV.

I asked Dr Davidson about the CD4 cells. I wanted to know whether the HIV actually destroyed them or just prevented the body from renewing them. He told me that only a few cells needed to be infected and then the others got the message and destroyed themselves. This is known as programmed cell destruction and isn't yet well understood. I asked him also whether there was anything I could do to improve my CD4 count. He explained to me how the mind works on the immune system via the hypothalamus which affects the pituitary gland causing it to release hormones which act on the immune system. He cited the instance of the woman who has had breast cancer and whose husband then dies. The breast cancer is liable to recur. He advised me to take plenty of rest and to avoid stress. A holiday could do good. He suggested I should get in touch with the Terrence Higgins Trust. They have a range of groups and activities which are aimed at promoting well-being. He also mentioned 'buddying'. This is where one is assigned a partner. The partner is not a conventional friend but rather someone in whom one can confide one's innermost thoughts feelings or fears. He thought I was in robust health. I confessed to him that I hadn't gone back to work. He said that if I didn't feel ready to go back it would probably knock me for six. I went and had an X-ray. It showed that the Pneumothorax had gone and my lung had reinflated.

Eva thinks I should give the letter to Dr Kapembwa. She says it gives him a free hand to try out any treatments he thinks fit. It also covers him legally should any of these treatments make me ill or even lead to my death. I'm still not sure. I don't want him to think I am deluding myself that I could be cured. I won't be seeing him for another month so I've got some more time to think about it.

Nine years ago, back in 1984, we took a house for the Summer down on the South Coast. This appeared at the time quite a risky venture. It was the first family holiday in fifteen years. The village is a quiet place where the well-heeled retire to. It is full of private roads with large houses; there are a few shops, a newsagent, chemist, general store, Post Office and a betting shop. You can get what you need for everyday purposes. We had a little house on a modern estate. The weather throughout the whole of August was really quite good. I had taken my bicycle down and it was a delight to pedal along the quiet country roads. You couldn't actually swim there that year as there was so much seaweed, but we drove a mile along the road to the next village where we bathed nearly every day off a rather painful, shingly beach. It wasn't an exciting holiday, but it was certainly enjoyable.

Alongside the general store and the newsagent was another important feature to the village, The Restaurant. This was more an institution, a day-care centre, where the elderly and very elderly met up for lunch for about five pounds a head. The food was excellent, the best of British cuisine. There was always a joint, steak and kidney pie, liver and bacon or fish. The restaurant wasn't licensed so you took your bottle of wine with you. Apart from preparing and cooking the food, serving, clearing away and washing up, Paddy entertained his visitors with gossip and chat. His mother, who was in her eighties, sat in the next room with the cash register singing. She would then come into the restaurant walking precariously in very high-heeled shoes and talk to the guests.

I struck up a bit of a friendship with Paddy and since then, whenever we fancy a trip to the coast, we set off down to The Restaurant. His mother has since died, but we always have a tremendous welcome from Paddy and a lovely meal. Several times I have gone to stay for a few days. I wait until the weather looks as though it is going to be good for a few days and then I drive down. I take a room in a hotel, but lunch is by courtesy of The Restaurant. Usually I'm lucky with the weather and spend my time sunning myself and swimming, but there have been times when it has rained and the wind has blown and it has seemed like winter.

The last Saturday in March the weather looked promising and my mother and I decided to have a trip down to the coast. This was the first day trip for me since I became ill and I felt anxious beforehand. My mother drove down. When we arrived, the sun was shining. We went for a drink and then on to Paddy's. We both enjoy his food. I had lamb and my mum had his steak and kidney. After lunch we drove along to Felpham and parked the car. We walked along the promenade in the direction of Bognor. The tide was in and the wind was off the sea. It was sunny, but very chilly. There is a little open train called James which runs the half mile between Butlins and the Regis Centre in Bognor. We got into the last carriage, Bluebell, and five minutes later we were in the centre of Bognor and looking round a little street market. We took the train back and then walked along to the Boat House Restaurant in Felpham for a cup of tea. As I looked at the sea, which was green and cold and quite rough, I wondered whether, if I immersed myself in it for twenty minutes, I might be cleansed of my infection. Probably I would just have died of cold. At four o'clock we set off home. I felt tired, but I drove back, I'm not going to be written off yet. The next two days I felt very weary again, but that may have been in part due to the clocks being put forward an hour.

March has flown past, what with my week in hospital and a week licking my wounds. I am nearly eleven stone now and there is no more news from the hospital which might cause concern. I have eaten and nursed myself back to comparative health. The mental aspect is far tougher. Life feels precarious. It is as though I have the sword of Damocles hanging over me.

The daffs are finishing now, but the trees are just starting to come into leaf and the forget-me-nots are out, the blue and the white. I had a pink forget-me-not once; it was a very pretty plant. The prunus trees have lost their blossom, but I saw a white flowering cherry in a garden in Temple Fortune. I had never seen one before.

The country has been mourning the death of two young toddlers, two-year-old James Bulger, who was murdered by two ten-year-olds; and three-year-old Jonathan Ball, victim of a terrorist's bomb in Warrington. This bombing, which also claimed the life of Tim Parry, caused particular anger and revulsion. All these deaths, James's in particular, have moved the whole country in a way I have never witnessed before. People everywhere have been drawn together, united in their horror and grief.

Part Five

At the end of January I had been brushing my teeth one evening when I managed to dislodge a filling in one of my upper teeth. It left what felt like a great chasm when I probed it with my tongue. Fortunately it didn't hurt. Having just been diagnosed as having TB, I thought I should check with the clinic before making arrangements to see my dentist. Dr Kapembwa advised me to wait a couple of weeks so my treatment could start to take effect.

Eventually, on 1st April, I had an appointment. My dentist had of course to be told. I explained to him that since I had last seen him, about six months ago, I had tested positive for HIV. I said that if he didn't feel comfortable treating me I would understand and go elsewhere. No hard feelings. I thought I would have my dental work also carried out at Northwick Park. If I were a dentist I'm not sure I would want to work on an HIV patient. A young man and recently married, he seemed to have no such misgivings. He immediately said that he thought it would be churlish to deny me treatment when he had already done so much work on me. I was apparently the first patient he had treated who admitted to being HIV positive.

He told his assistant and they took extra precautions. He always wears gloves, but he also used a mask as did his assistant who, in addition, put on eye protectors. He told her to confine herself to one area which they could swab down afterwards. He decided not to use the fast drill because of the cloud of vapour it produced. He seemed genuinely interested in my condition and asked me a lot of questions which I found difficult to answer with the drill and his mirror in my mouth. When he had finished he suggested that in the future I should come at the end of the day so that they would have time to swab everything down properly. He talked about the dangers of cross-infection and about the fragility of the HIV virus compared with hepatitis B which can apparently live for thirty-six hours outside the human body and causes more deaths than HIV. He didn't seem unduly worried and explained that all the equipment was autoclaved.

The rain was still pelting down outside when I left and the traffic was dreadful. I felt very sad. He had been very positive about continuing to treat me, he had shown interest and he had been kind. I just didn't want to be treated any differently from normal. Certainly the precautions he took were wise, as was his suggestion to treat me at the end of the day, but I couldn't help feeling a bit like a leper.

I drove back to Edgware. Last Summer my hi-fi had started making strange rustling noises. I took it to a dealer who checked it out and pronounced the speakers dead. I had agonised for months over what to do. I could just buy a new pair of speakers and attach them to the amplifier, but that was also eighteen years old and might give up at any moment, or I could buy a new system. In the end I decided on the latter course of action. Sopping wet, I arrived at the shop with my old amp and tuner which were also dripping with water. They offered me a very good deal and I came away pleased with the transaction. When I got home I removed the new system from its boxes and proceeded to set it up. This proved more complicated than I had anticipated, what with all the plugs and wires which needed to be stripped. I doubted my ability to do it and felt very fed up. I thought to myself: 'What am I doing buying a new hi-fi system when I'm going to die any minute?' I also remembered that Howard had bought himself a system only months before he died. I bent the aerial pin and both the aerial and my old turntable had the wrong connectors for the new system. The CD player had a fault and wouldn't play properly either. I was really down in the dumps and the rain continued to pour down.

The next day, by contrast, was a beautiful sunny day. I went back to the shop with my problems. They sorted me out. I came back to the flat and, feeling fresher than the evening before, methodically set about wiring it all up, it took a couple of hours, but it all worked fine. I haven't any great confidence in my practical skills so I was delighted. I recognised also that I had done the right thing by buying it. Death may be just around the corner for any one of us, but you cannot allow that fact to prevent you from getting on with your life.

It was that day too that the reports appeared in the media about AZT. It does not delay the onset of AIDS for HIV patients though it does prolong life for people with AIDS. The shares of the Wellcome

Foundation had fallen more than fifty pence. I was interested in the news and followed the bulletins throughout the day, but my interest in it seemed somehow detached, as if I were untouched by the news. Half way through the afternoon I realised I had forgotten to take my AZT. I quickly put that right. I couldn't help feeling that this report was perhaps a blessing in disguise. If AZT really were a wonder drug why did people continue to die? Now if AZT were shown to be of no value whatsoever for people with HIV it meant there was nothing to give them at all. This would renew the search for an effective drug and perhaps spur researchers on in their efforts to find something new, something which worked. It seemed good too that it had made front page headlines in the quality newspapers. I felt quite hopeful.

I went out to get *The Independent* and *The Times*. What would they have to say?

The three-year-old Anglo-French trial, Concorde, involving one thousand seven hundred participants showed that treatment with AZT failed to protect healthy HIV positive people from developing AIDS. The trial did identify a short-term benefit in the early stages of the study, but that did not last. These preliminary results were expected to reflect the final outcome of the trial. They do not affect the benefit of giving the drug to people with AIDS, who can extend their lives by an average of about nine months or more with treatment.

AIDS researchers are hoping that treatment for HIV using two or more drugs will prove more effective. The virus mutates so rapidly in the body that it soon develops strains resistant to AZT. Using two or more drugs makes this more difficult.

To hijack a human cell and turn it into a virus factory, the virus needs to copy itself into the human DNA. The transformation is orchestrated by an enzyme, reverse transcriptase, which builds up in long chains of the DNA carrying the viral genes. AZT, known as a chain terminator, attempts to stop the enzyme making the long chain. It is this ability that is now in serious doubt after the Concorde study. It is hoped that the virus's ability to copy itself into the DNA can be better undermined in combination.

A new drugs trial, Delta, will explore the benefits of using AZT in conjunction with ddI or ddC. They work in a similar way to AZT by blocking the vital enzyme that HIV needs for replication.

Two alternatives to drugs are aimed at boosting the body's own defences against HIV before the virus can destroy the vital cells of the immune system.

There is a 'therapeutic vaccine' based on one of the proteins in the virus, developed by British Biotechnology Group based in Oxford. The aim of this genetically engineered protein, p24-VLP, is to stimulate the body's immune system to recognise this viral protein, reverse transcriptase, and attack it, thereby keeping virus replication in check.

Another approach is to take the natural antibodies produced by healthy HIV positive people and infuse them into patients with AIDS. This passive immunisation has produced promising preliminary results.

Scientists have found that the virus is more active in the early stages of infection than had previously been believed. Rather than lying dormant in the 'latent' stage between infection and the onset of AIDS HIV has been found to be present in large quantities in the lymph glands, where it is active throughout the latency period. Also an extraordinarily large number of blood cells of the type favoured by HIV are found to be infected from an early stage. These two facts call for early treatment of HIV infection hitting the virus hard in its early stages.

It was felt that what has happened this week will probably advance, rather than set back, the search for an AIDS cure. It was not considered to be an unconquerable virus.

I lapped up all this information and felt quite excited. Here at last were some new ideas. It was Good Friday or God's Friday, as I had heard on the radio that morning, and I listened to *The Morning Worship* with the Bishop of Southwark. I was very moved to hear again the story of the Crucifixion. One man had laid down His life to save the world. People had jeered at Him and said that He couldn't even save himself. The sky had turned dark and at the moment of death He had felt abandoned and cried out:

"My God, my God, why hast thou forsaken me?"

After the Easter holiday I resolved that I would ask Dr Kapembwa to add ddI to my treatment. I also wanted to explore the genetically engineered protein p24-VLP. That sounded really promising.

I saw this as the start of my own individual medical trials. Okay, so I could only save thirteen million people and there was a degree of self-interest, but at least it was a start. Maybe I couldn't save anyone at all, not even myself, but I was going to try and I knew I had nothing to lose. Dr Kapembwa would have to accommodate me in this, it gave an important new meaning and purpose to my post-HIV life. If the worst came to the worst I knew that at least I would never be abandoned.

When I thought about the research which was being done I always wondered how many of the researchers were HIV positive or had AIDS. Very few, if any, I supposed.

There was another dimension which I knew I would be foolish to ignore. When reason and science fail and have to be abandoned we can always be guided by the voice within us, which emerges from deep within the psyche. It contains within it the whole body of experience since life began, the whole of the human condition. This was potentially the most powerful resource of all. It alone leads us to the truth and would also hold the answer to my problem if I could only hear and interpret that voice, I thought of Blake:

> Hear the voice of the Bard
> Who present, past and future sees.
> Whose ears have heard
> The Holy Word
> That walked among the ancient trees.
>
> Calling the lapsed soul
> And weeping in the evening dew.

For whatever reason this infection had been wished on me, I felt a commitment to it and, whether I liked it or not, I was involved and I was prepared to spend the rest of my life fighting it. Clearly the virus wasn't susceptible to compromise. I wanted to be involved with the research. I was not a medical or scientific man, but I had the virus. I was living with it every day in my body. I felt that I could recognise intuitively more readily than scientists, medics or researchers what would fight off my infection in my body. I knew I was on my own with only my intuition to guide me.

Intuition told me also that I had been infected round about 1979. Back in the hospital in December I had wondered about this. Now I knew, I didn't need to ring Phil or John. The pieces of the jigsaw, which for so many years I had struggled with, just fell into place. The picture was nearly complete. Nor had I been asymptomatic. There had been minor physical ailments like the migraine that I had never had before, and the chicken pox, but these were insignificant. For nine years I had had psychological problems. I had thought I was having a breakdown and couldn't understand why. Eva was the only person I ever confided in. Week in, week out, for years I had gone to see her with the same message: "What is wrong with me?" Her answer was always the same: "You're depressed". I had been angry with her. I knew there was no reason for me to be depressed, but I knew I didn't feel right and I spent hours just crying. Several times I had said to her, "I feel like I've got a virus in my brain." I felt like an unreal player in an unreal world, an observer from a distant planet. I thought perhaps I had had a slight stroke. I wasn't focused at all and I felt I was going mad. I seemed to have sunk down into my own unconscious and my world had become the unconscious world. I could see and understand what other people were blind to, but I had lost the ability to function in the real world. I had even threatened to commit myself, saying: "We'll see who is mad." I have heard it suggested that madness is just an extreme form of sanity and from my experience I would certainly endorse that view. Later on I had started drinking heavily. It was the only time I felt at one with myself and the world. In 1988, when my father got sick and I was driving down to Sutton every other day to visit him in hospital, I did manage to focus myself better, and since then I've not been so bad. In fact the AZT seems to have helped.

Eleanor was the only person who had picked up unconsciously on this malfunctioning, and had taken to ringing me every day to ask if I was all right or how I was. The daily intrusion of these phone calls had irritated me immensely at the time. It was possibly also the reason why I hadn't enjoyed my holidays. I just didn't feel safe away from my flat. For a while I had even found it an ordeal to go and post a letter. It was like going out into a hostile world.

It felt desperately unfair that what I had done fourteen years ago in innocence, and certainly ignorance, should be visited on me now at the age of forty-one when I was quite a different person in quite a different stage of my life. In a way also it had blighted the last. fourteen years. I had not been myself. It also seemed unfair that this illness was targeting a group of people who had had to confront hostility and prejudice all their lives.

As I said at the outset my plan had been not to test unless I felt I needed to, if I became ill. My expectation was that that would then be the last stage of the infection and my final illness. In that way I avoided the anxiety as to when I would get sick. So at the end of November when I tested positive and was taken to hospital I imagined that I would be dead by now. However, with the treatment I have received my health has improved. Yesterday I went for a four mile hike on the North Downs and the only ill effect was that my ankles ached a little. I realise now that I have to concentrate on living with AIDS instead of dying from AIDS. This represents a huge shift in emphasis.

I am glad I am still alive. I have nearly had another Spring and perhaps it may not be my last. I have resolved that there should be as much beauty in my life as possible. There was music to be listened to, poetry to be read. The significance of the hi-fi was that it allowed the music back into my life. If I died tomorrow it had already provided enjoyment for me and proved its worth. I thought of Plato's 'single science, which is the science of beauty everywhere' and Keats:

> Beauty is Truth, Truth Beauty, that is all
> Ye know on earth, and all ye need to know.

I went to church on Easter Day, not in the hope of being cured. I don't subscribe to that sort of thing, nor of being saved, that's up to God, but because I wanted to go. Easter is the most important day in the church calendar. I would have preferred to have gone to the morning service when the church is full, but this wasn't really possible. By the time I have taken my twelve tablets to start the day and had a cup of tea, my fluid intake has been so great that I spend the morning going to the toilet. We went to Evensong instead. The flowers in the church were beautiful. I think people were probably flexing their muscles ready for the flower festival later in the year. There were one or two changes. The gold cross on the altar table had gone and another font had appeared in the central aisle. There were only about twenty people there. I fumbled about with the Common

Prayer trying to follow the Order of Service, but the words came back to me. We sang a couple of hymns which I didn't know. I suppose they had sung the best Easter hymns in the Morning Service. We said prayers and forty minutes later it was over. After the service the vicar came up to talk to me. He told me the story of the 'new' font. Shortly after he joined the parish in 1983 he received a letter from the Wantage Sisters at St Mary's Home in Alton. They wondered whether he would like to have the font back. It had been loaned to them in 1868 and they had now finished with it. The cross had been removed when the altar table had been moved away from the front wall of the church. I think that this was a mistake. The cross had always been the focal point.

A couple of days later our neighbours, Peter and Barbara, went away for a few days, taking the children with them, I suppose, unless they had left them bound and gagged in the attic with just a mouldy crust of bread. It strikes me that this is a wholly appropriate way to deal with children. Anyway, whether or not they left the children behind they did leave the cats. Another neighbour down the road came to feed them twice a day, but they spent a lot of time with us in the garden. At night they settled down together on our front porch. They were obviously missing Peter and Barbara and every evening they sat in front of the house looking down the road, waiting for their car. One evening I went out and Tiger trotted up shouting for attention. I sat down on the front step and she hopped onto my lap. She circled round a few times and then settled down in a frenzy of ecstasy purring like a little generator. I hadn't noticed that Soldier had sidled up to us. He was lonely too. I stretched out my hand to him for him to sniff and then he let me stroke him. I had never dreamt that he would allow me to and I felt privileged. This was all too much for Tiger. That most affectionate little creature hissed at him. She lay in my lap growling. He walked round to the other side of me and she lashed out at him with her claws and then shot off in high dudgeon. I realised now why Soldier was wary and usually held back. It was easy to see who was top dog here.

I had a big row with my mother over something which was, on the face of it, very trivial (four pork chops). I thought we had agreed that I was going to cook them, not that I particularly wanted to. Then she changed her mind and wanted to cook them herself, having obviously decided, without consulting me, that I wasn't up to it. I was cross, it seemed like she was writing me off and dismissing this small contribution that I was able to make. I said crossly to her that I wasn't dead yet. She was furious with me, but the rebuke was too vehement and I ended up feeling completely crushed and withdrew into myself.

She had been away for a few days staying with Eleanor and she must have been aware of the contrast on her return, if only unconsciously. She has a nice house and garden and a nice car. She has a cat, two goldfish and a job she is married to. Here was I with this wretched infection which I had contracted through sex, homosexual sex at that. I was the one causing her the problems, perhaps I always had.

I felt she was angry with me and was growing weary of me. I already knew how difficult she was finding it to deal with the reality of my infection. I wasn't ever going to be cured; there was nothing that would help against the tiredness, apart from my tablets, not even Lucozade. I felt also she was starting to infantilise me. It was an impossibly difficult situation for any mother.

I resolved not to interfere in the cooking and to try to protect her from certain aspects of my illness, particularly the hopelessness. I decided it was time for me to come back to Stanmore. The time we were spending together wasn't doing either of us any good. When I was there she abandoned her friends and her day revolved around caring for me. I wasn't ungrateful, but despite the long walks we took every afternoon I was getting bored. I needed my own things around me and I was missing my friends.

I spent most of that week reading John Langone's excellent book *AIDS the facts*. It was hard work and slow-going, but I believe in knowing the enemy and I think I have understood quite a lot. It seems, from what I have read, that I have a maximum of two years left.

I decided that I wanted to find out what the current state of research was and wondered how I could obtain such information. I phoned the National AIDS Helpline who suggested I should get in touch with the National AIDS Manual (NAM). They produce an annual publication, which costs about two hundred and twenty-five pounds, which contains up-to-date information about all the most recent trials and treatments. I rang. They were ever so helpful.

They have a monthly treatment update which was started last November which they are prepared to send free of charge to individuals. The girl said she would send me all the back issues.

I heard it on the radio first at about twenty to eight in the morning. Fifteen of the world's top pharmaceutical companies (six American and nine European) are going to pool their resources to try to find a cure for AIDS. This followed the realisation by scientists that no single drug will combat HIV and that viral resistance will develop against any compound. They will collaborate by swapping information on drugs that have been developed, provide samples for laboratory and clinical trial work, and keep each other informed about development techniques. There were already many more compounds available which were effective against HIV. What they had to find was the right combination of these drugs. The stimulus for this had, of course, been the disappointing outcome of the Concorde trial. The spokesman said that there were many things which worked well in the test-tube and that we could expect new combinations of drugs to appear in a matter of months. I think he said that there were about ninety anti-HIV drugs which had now been developed.

I resolved to sit tight and wait. There would be no holiday in Greece, which I had been planning and where I might get a potentially lethal infection. I remembered that Howard had died of salmonella and that I had thought he had picked it up in Tunisia a few months before he died. There would be no return to work where the stress might worsen my condition. I just had to be patient and hope that something would turn up.

I decided that it was time to start reviewing my options, one of which was to apply for early retirement on medical grounds. I had been told to avoid stress so how could I seriously contemplate going back to that school? I knew that Dr Segal would back me up. I rang up LAGER (Lesbian and Gay Employment Rights) and spoke to Phil Greasley, who was most painstaking with the advice he gave me. I wanted to know whether I should phone the County Council myself to inquire or ask my union to act on my behalf. Should I disclose the fact that I had AIDS? He advised me to ring the union first and advised me not to say that I had AIDS. He didn't know whether Hertfordshire had an HIV policy.

I rang the union and spoke to Gwen Mansfield, who guided me through the whole procedure. She confirmed that I had one hundred days on full-pay and worked out that that would run out in May. Then I would go onto half-pay for a further hundred days plus Statutory Sick Pay. When the Statutory Sick Pay ran out after a few weeks I would be entitled to Invalidity Benefit from the DHSS. She worked out that I would receive £6,900 per year and a lump sum of around £20,000. She advised me to start my application at the end of May. She was very helpful and also very kind, but after I had spoken to her I felt rotten. So this was it, the end of my working life. I decided that I would try to delay as long as possible my decision about my job. I didn't want to join the scrap-heap yet. That school was starting to seem more attractive, but I didn't want to be carried out of it in a box. Gwen had given me all the information I wanted and so I didn't need to phone the County Council.

But how could I live off £6,900 a year? I didn't want to give up my flat or my car. The only concession I was prepared to make was to give up eating fillet steak. However, I knew that the basis for any decision I made must not be financial, I had to decide what was best for my health. If that meant giving up work, so be it.

The day before my next appointment I received the first six issues of the Treatment Update from NAM. I sat down and read through the first one. The reading I had done enabled me to understand and make sense of the articles. They were just what I wanted. It was interesting to find out about the research and developments, treatments and trials, and it was heartening to know that something was going on. There was one paragraph in particular which caught my attention and which I read over and over again. There was a new treatment, known as convergent combination therapy, which seemed to work in laboratory studies. It appeared that there was a limit to the number of reverse transcriptase mutations which the virus could develop and remain fully functioning. Simultaneous mutations conferring resistance to AZT, ddI and a non-nucleoside reverse transcriptase inhibitor like nevirapine appeared to shut the virus down. It could neither replicate nor infect new cells. At last there was something that worked, theoretically at least in the test-tube, though it was not known whether it was effective, or even safe, in human beings.

I recalled Jung's theory of synchronicity. This is described as 'when events coinciding in time and space also have meaningful psychological connections' in the 'Critical Dictionary of Jungian Analysis' by Samuels, Shorter and Plaut. Some would call it coincidence, others the hand of God. It seemed to me like the intervention of a higher power I felt that there was a message in it for me.

There had been the disappointing outcome of the Concorde trial, the decision by the pharmaceutical companies to pool their resources and now this, convergent combination therapy. It was the third and most remarkable instance of synchronicity. Someone seemed to be wanting me to survive and I started thinking that maybe I wouldn't die of AIDS after all.

I had a very long session with Dr Kapembwa the next time I saw him. As I walked into his consulting room there were tears in my eyes. I think that Thursday afternoon is probably the HIV clinic, but I've never asked and no one has ever said anything. There are certainly very few people there, sometimes no one at all. However, on a few occasions I have seen one gentleman. He is middle-aged, in his fifties perhaps. I would guess he was a manual worker from his large, solid frame, big hands and jeans. He comes with a younger chap who pushes his wheelchair. He is obviously very sick and he just sits and looks straight ahead. He was there again, but this time he was far worse. He had lost a lot of weight and I could see his bones through his skin. He sat slumped in the wheelchair with his chin resting on his chest. I thought he might die at any moment, and I kept looking to see if he was still breathing. When they left the waiting room I started to cry. I felt so helpless, had wanted to take his hand, to say "hello", to give him a kiss, but I hadn't liked to. Dr Kapembwa was very kind to him. I never saw him again.

At last Dr Kapembwa had received the sensitivities. The Xenopi was sensitive to Rifampicin, but not to Isoniazid or Pyrazinamide, or only partially so. As I seemed to be doing well on my present treatment he did not propose changing my drugs. He had, however, asked for further sensitivities to be done with some second-line drugs.

He had a good look at me and said I had a good haemoglobin. I wasn't sure what that was, but it sounded like a compliment and so I thanked him.

I gave him my letter, explaining that I had written it over a month ago, but because of recent developments it seemed even more relevant now. He sat and read it. He turned and looked at me. He said he felt flattered, that he saw it as a challenge, that he had never had a letter like that before from a patient. He actually seemed quite moved by the trouble I had obviously taken over it and by its content, I felt pleased that I had decided to give it to him.

Before my appointment I had resolved, in the light of the results of the Concorde trial, press reports and what I had read in the first Treatment Update, that the time had come to review my treatment for the HIV. It seemed unlikely that monotherapy with AZT could defeat the virus since it mutates and forms resistance to any single drug. However, there seemed to be evidence that the antiviral drugs might work better in combination. The first objective had to be to try to disable the virus and stop it replicating before more damage was done to the immune system. I told Dr Kapembwa about what I had read and how simultaneous mutations in response to AZT, ddI and nevirapine appeared to shut the virus down and stop it replicating. I don't know if he already knew about this, but he didn't seem very excited. I suppose he has seen many promising ideas fail over the last years.

I wanted to go for broke. My CD4 count was low and there was everything to play for and nothing to lose. Dr Kapembwa is a cautious man, as befits a doctor. I am not. I didn't know how he would react to my proposal to start combination therapy. I thought he would probably be content to let me continue with the AZT, but I knew that this would never be enough to defeat the virus. I think that basically he agreed with what I had written and endorsed the synergistic effect of two or more drugs. I explained how important it was to me, how it gave my life a new purpose, but I knew I was beholden to him. He would have to monitor me, measure my CD4 count and viral antigen levels.

He started talking about the Delta trial, but I pointed out that my CD4 count was so low that there was no time to lose, I wanted to start immediately. My plan was to start the ddI straight away and then, a month later, if I had had no adverse reaction to it to add nevirapine. Apparently AZT is the only licensed drug for HIV in this country and he would have to approach the drug company directly and request the ddI under the named patient scheme from Bristol-Myers Squibb. He agreed to do this, but asked me to put my request in writing. I was to go back the following Thursday with my letter; it also gave him time to think about it. I wanted his blessing, but I wasn't sure whether I had it and I don't think he knew either.

That day Lesley's car was stolen from outside her office. It was only a year ago that someone had broken into my car and taken the radio. It had been in my garage, locked, I could remember how I had felt and this was worse, I think that I was sympathetic, but I was feeling very excited.

I was consumed by my plan and there was so much more reading that I had to do in order to get a clearer picture. Again I started feeling I was on my own. This was uncharted ground and I felt apprehensive. Apart from Dr Kapembwa there was no one I knew who understood enough to talk it over with. My Uncle David was back in Florida. Somehow I had to find the confidence to implement my plan. I had taken the first step, but I knew there would be setbacks. My trial was about to begin. I had to be determined and, above all, had to learn to be patient and I had to look after myself.

At the weekend I went on reading the Treatment Updates and discovered that the next big American trial, which is to start in July, will study the effects of combination therapy using those drugs which I had read about. I decided to write some letters to people whose names I had read in connection with research. First of all there were Professor Robert Gallo and Professor Luc Montagnier. They had been the first two to discover the virus back in 1983 and were probably ahead of the competition in the research field. Gallo works at the National Cancer Institute in Maryland and Montagnier is at the Pasteur Institute in Paris. Then there was Professor Margaret Fischl at the University of Miami School of Medicine. She was involved in the American trials and had strong views about combination therapy. I wrote also to Dr Linda Distlerath whose name I had seen in the Independent. She works with the pharmaceutical company, Merck, which initiated the collaboration between companies to find a cure. Finally I wrote to Dr Kevin Cahill, a personal friend of Eva, who practises in New York and who is very interested in HIV infection. They all got the same letter apart from Montagnier who had an extra paragraph in French. I got the addresses from the French and

American embassies and put the letters in the post. I wonder if I'll have any replies.

Monday evening was Capital Radio and Revision Line. This is a service which is offered in conjunction with Letts. It is not broadcast on air, but children who are revising for some exams can ring in and speak to a subject specialist for advice. It was set up many years ago when Lesley was working at Capital. In fact, she had run it for a number of years. It was just two hours in the evening once a year and it was well-paid.

I felt terribly apprehensive all day. I had used the toilet three times by half past nine and felt tired. Finally I fell asleep in the afternoon. I went round to Maria's house at five o'clock for a cup of tea and then at six we set off together for Watford Junction Station. We arrived at Capital about three minutes to seven, acknowledged the other members of the team, people I only see once a year and whose names I always forget. Then the phones started ringing. We were very busy. The enquiries all tend to be similar. The children want to revise, but don't know how to go about it. They are grateful for the advice they receive and you feel that they will go off and do some work. We were fed with wine and sandwiches. I felt fine, like I had never been ill. At the end, when we came away I was so pleased I had managed and managed so well, and had some pasta with Maria and her husband, Ed, that when we got back and I got into my flat at about a quarter to midnight, I started thinking perhaps I would be able to go back to work.

Someone else was obviously thinking the same thing for on Tuesday evening I had a phone call from Geoff, my headmaster. He asked me how I was and I told him I was doing all right. I mentioned to him the Xenopi and the shadow on my lung. The reason he had rung was because he was aware that my hundred days of full-pay were running out. He had approached a couple of the governors to see whether they could do anything to extend this. It depended naturally on when I might be able to return to work. He wanted to get in touch with my GP to see how I was doing. I told him that I was hoping to return in September, but that depended largely on my medication. The antibiotics hit my stomach so hard that I spent half the morning on the toilet. I told him I would ask Dr Kapembwa to drop him a line about me.

This seemed jolly decent of him. He had joined our school under two years ago and this was the first time he had willingly spoken to me. Naturally, I hadn't liked him much, but this phone call raised him in my estimation. I even felt I would like to come clean with him and tell him about the HIV, but I didn't feel I knew him well enough. This was a shame; it would have made life easier.

I went back to the clinic the following Thursday armed with my letter, twenty-four hours' worth of urine and another long list of things to say. The urine was to be used to monitor the shadow on my lung. The tumour had been described as carcenoid and they were going to monitor the hormone levels in my body. I weighed in at just over eleven stone.

I started apologising to Dr Kapembwa in case he felt that I had been trying to interfere in my treatment. I pointed out that people probably react differently on discovering they are HIV positive. My way of dealing with the infection was to find out everything I could about the virus and its mechanisms and to read about all the treatments and trials. Then, of course, I drew conclusions and wanted to make decisions on the basis of what I had read. It really just showed how much better I was feeling and that I wasn't prepared to lie down and let this beat me.

However, the bottom line was that I would not embark on any course of treatment if I didn't have his blessing, and if he thought that monotherapy with AZT was the best course of action for the time being, that was what I would do.

He felt that I was doing well on the AZT, that I was benefiting from it and still improving. He told me that the first mutations of the virus are only detectable after six months, and he felt I should continue with it at least until then. Nor did he want to jeopardise the treatment of the Xenopi, which seemed to be responding so well, by introducing new drugs. He decided to stop the Pyrazinamide as the Xenopi was not sensitive to it and it seemed to hit my stomach so hard.

He said that he had no ethical problem with combination therapy; there was another patient in the clinic who was on it. We would keep it in mind and review my treatment periodically. If he found that my response to AZT declined it would be a real option.

He talked about the limited reliability of the CD4 count as a surrogate marker. There is one patient in the clinic whose CD4 count is nil and yet, apart from herpes, he has had no opportunistic infections and is the fittest HIV patient that Dr Kapembwa sees. However, a combination of AZT and ddI did seem to raise and sustain the CD4 count. When pressed he told me that his own count was six hundred and fifty which is at the lower end of the range for non-HIV people.

I think he is marvellous. He is not only prepared to discuss all the different options with me and to explain things I don't understand, but seems to enjoy doing so. He said I had put a lot of thought into my notes.

I had a quick word with Karen before I came away. She looked overworked and fed up, but she said that they all enjoyed my visits, that I cheered them up. But I knew how much my visits and all the clinic staff helped me and how good they made me feel.

I was happy with what we had decided, but perhaps a little disappointed. It did make sense. My medical trial would have to wait a while. I think I was relieved. I really wasn't keen to experience the side-effects of ddI, but when it was necessary I knew I would take it.

What I have realised from this episode is that I am keen to start combination therapy when it is appropriate to do so. It is the only hope of defeating the virus.

It is the end of April. The weather hasn't been great, but I have been for a number of walks. I've spent most of this month reading and writing. My writing is more important to me than anything, more important than my health or even death. It is in a sense my weapon against the virus and everything else has become subsidiary to it. In consequence other areas of my life have been neglected. This isn't good and I should go out more and visit friends, but I have felt compelled to understand about my infection and to contain it in my mind. Then perhaps it won't seem so frightening.

Since last November I have confronted daily the prospect of my death. I don't want it and I am still quite scared, but slowly I am beginning to come to terms with the idea of it. It strikes me that even if I were somehow to survive AIDS it isn't as if I am securing everlasting life for myself, so what does it really matter when I die, now or in twenty years? My mother and sister, who depend on me, would miss me as would my friends, no doubt, but the lovers I have had have deserted me and I am not going to have children or grandchildren. All this seems to diminish my worth as a human being in my own eyes. There are many others who have a more urgent claim to life. I just want to finish my writing. I see it as perhaps my one and only achievement. It is, I suppose, my response to my illness, a measure of self-preservation, an attempt to leave behind something of myself for the people I loved, for the world, something rather more than a letter saying: 'I loved you'. It is a testimony to and an assertion of the fact that I existed.

There are several thoughts still unresolved in my mind and Eva has had her hands full with me this month. Sometimes I feel that I owe everything I have become to her. There is a real sense in which I am not ill. Even as I am contemplating my death I am considering going back to work. This is complicated and confusing. Then again, how would I cope if a cure were found in time to save me? It would take me a long time to deal with that about-turn, it might be harder than what I've already been through. I would have to find a meaning and purpose in my life beyond what I have found so far. It is perhaps easier to die now.

Sometimes I just sit in the garden. Looking at the flowers and shrubs and trees isn't enough anymore. I need to touch them and confide in them. Sometimes as I sit there I can feel my eyes heavy with tears. It is all too beautiful to leave behind and my faith isn't strong enough.

Part Six

I had been reading an article in the NAM Treatment Update by a chap who had tested positive in 1986 with a CD4 count of one hundred. After treatment with AZT his count had risen to five hundred. I had had blood taken at the end of April and I was waiting anxiously to see whether my count had risen again and by what margin. I was hoping for one hundred if not more. I phoned up the clinic and Anne went away to check in my file. Ninety-two. I was disappointed. I felt so much fitter than in February when I last had my blood taken that I was sure that the count would have rocketed up. It seemed like the benefit I was receiving from the AZT was reaching a peak, and a very small peak at that. I knew from what Dr Kapembwa had said and from what I had read that the count is not a reliable indicator of clinical status, but I had nothing else to hang on to. One thing, however, is certain: the lower the count the greater the likelihood of opportunistic infections and mortality. For me it was a measure of how secure life was.

My sister has always been marvellously uncensorious. I remember when, many years ago, I had told her I was homosexual, she responded with a single word: "Oh" and never mentioned it again. It made no difference to her, and why should it, I was still her brother.

Our relationship hadn't been so good since our father had died. I felt she looked to me to provide the love and affection which she was wont to receive from him. I don't think she was aware of it, but I knew I couldn't supply what she was looking for and that any attempt to do so would fail. It felt like an unfair expectation on her part and also meant that she overlooked what I could still offer her as a brother. When I told her I was HIV positive, she remained absolutely calm and I was able to discuss sensibly with her whether or not to tell my mother.

I had planned to go and visit her at the beginning of March, but it was then that I had been called back into hospital for my tests. I hadn't been up to see her for nearly five years. Since my father had died there had seemed to be so little time. I was trying to visit my mother frequently and what time I had left in the holidays I needed for myself. I had decided not to take the car as I felt the long drive would be tiring so I had bought a ticket for the coach. It left Golders Green at two o'clock, and arrived in Dewsbury at five. I don't think I could have driven it any faster.

I was feeling a bit apprehensive for many reasons. I still wasn't sleeping well, my bowels, though predictable, needed to express themselves sometimes several times in the morning and I find that Eleanor can be somewhat intimidating. She is very positive and can be rather sharp. This makes me feel uncomfortable and also undermines my confidence so that I start to make silly mistakes I feel she is laughing at. I feel I have to watch very carefully everything I do or say. Having said all this, I love her dearly and was thrilled to be going to visit her again.

It was a hot sunny day and travelling upstairs in the coach with four seats to myself I had a wonderful view. Unfortunately, we hit very heavy traffic as soon as we joined the motorway and became part of the Friday afternoon crawl to escape from London. We must have lost about three quarters of an hour in the first hour, but I didn't care, it wasn't my responsibility. I just looked out of the window; drank beakers of tea that a hostess, obviously a Northern girl, brought and dozed. You don't have to get very far from London to be in the countryside. The light that afternoon was quite remarkable. Normally I never see fields, let alone emerald green fields or fields with sheep or cows in. I was astonished at how much countryside there is still left. The fields and the woods were almost uninterrupted for the next two hundred miles. Not far from Dewsbury we passed Markham colliery. There didn't seem to be any signs of life at first and I assumed that it had been closed down, but then I saw some trucks transporting coal to great reserves on the other side of the motorway. I suppose the activity was underground.

We were about half an hour late arriving in Dewsbury coach station and Eleanor was already there waiting for me in her spotted jeans. She's forty-six now, but looks much younger. She has retained an almost youthful quality. I wish she would get herself a man. She enjoys the company of men and I don't want her to end up alone. What struck me immediately as we were driving back to Eleanor's house was the different style of building, the Yorkshire stone-faced buildings and the dry-stone walls. It makes everything look darker than down in the South.

She lives in a terraced house which seems small from the outside. However, like the Tardis, there is plenty of room inside: a lounge, a dining room and three bedrooms. Behind the house is a garden with a lawn and flower beds and behind that some shrubs including a beautiful yellow broom, and a garage which you approach from the road behind. It is quiet, civilised, peaceful.

The cat came out to greet us and let me give him a fleeting stroke. We sat in the back garden and had a cup of tea. It was still gloriously hot in the sun. After *The Six o'clock News* my sister went upstairs to change and we walked down to a local Italian restaurant of some renown. It is the noisiest, liveliest, place I have ever eaten in. You can hardly hear yourself think, but it is great fun. I had what I always have, beef stroganoff, and she had veal and we shared a carafe of white wine. We ate well and I felt my long journey had already been justified. I slept very poorly that night. The sun had been shining into the back bedroom all afternoon and I was too hot.

In the morning she went out shopping while I attended to my toilet and then we had coffee. At the front the house overlooks the library, which is a very handsome stone building where the cat can frequently be seen disappearing into the bushes or shooting up trees. I decided to go for a little walk by myself. I walked round the library and came to the old cemetery with its chapel of rest, now boarded up. I walked among the graves. The earliest I saw was 1869. I looked at the inscriptions on the tombstones and was shocked at the number of children who had died before the age of ten and also the number who had died in infancy. I hadn't realised how high infant mortality was in those days. In one grave were buried two children, brother and sister, and with them two more whom the parents had then adopted. In another grave were two women. One had died in 1870 and the other, the second wife, had died in 1873. There was no mention of the husband of these two women and I wondered where and with whom he had found his final resting place. I resolved that, if I had time, I would go back with my note-book, and write down some of the verses and inscriptions. Unfortunately I didn't get the opportunity.

At about half past twelve we drove into Halifax where I had a substantial steak and kidney lunch in Harvey's, the departmental store. We wandered round the shops and went into the Coop, where I discovered a rather nice, mulberry-coloured lightweight summer jacket, reduced by ten pounds, which I bought. I was feeling very tired by now and rather light-headed because of lack of sleep and so we went into the Piece Hall and I found a bench in the sun where I sat and recovered my energy.

From the Middle Ages wool was the mainstay of Halifax's prosperity and was dried in the fields on wooden frames or tenters (hence the expression 'on tenterhooks'). On 1st January 1779 the Piece Hall was opened as a meeting place in which to sell 'pieces' of cloth. There are three hundred and fifteen rooms on three levels. Set around an enormous courtyard, the classical design incorporates an arcade of semi-circular arches, a gallery of square columns and a continuous gallery on the top floor. With the coming of the Industrial Revolution the cottage industries went into decline and from 1867 for the next hundred years the hall was used as a fish, fruit and vegetable market. Barely saved from demolition in 1972, it was reopened in 1976. No longer trading in cloth, there are gift and craft shops, an art gallery and industrial museum, weekly markets and public events.

We climbed up to the top floor and started looking in the various little shops. There are all sorts of bric-a-brac and souvenirs, but there is also a lot of skilled craftsmanship and we went into a wood shop where a young man was busy turning bowls and vases on his lathe. I spotted a very pretty little vase made of spalted beech. He explained to us that if you wait for the wood to start to rot it develops the interesting colours and patterns like the ones on the vase. Wait too long and the wood turns spongy. I bought the vase for my mother. It is delightful. In another shop, the herb emporium, I also bought her a little jar of acacia blossom honey and a packet of Assam tea bags by Taylors of Harrogate. Walking on round Eleanor spotted a second-hand book she had been looking for which is now out of print. We settled down to a cup of tea and then went home.

I slept a little that night, about four hours, and woke up feeling refreshed. I was still upstairs taking my tablets and drinking my tea when she reappeared. She had a migraine and was going to lie down.

Since she was a child she has suffered from severe migraines, flashing lights, nausea, the lot. When she was younger they used to put her out of action for a couple of days. Now they are not so severe, but still unpleasant. I got up and made my breakfast and took her a cup of tea. At about half past nine she came back downstairs and sat in the lounge. She looks strange when she has a migraine – rather like a psychopath, I thought. I got dressed and decided to go out and leave her undisturbed.

I walked down into town and decided to get some money from the machine outside the bank. It was no great surprise to discover that the machines are no more reliable there than elsewhere. 'Sorry, there is a fault'. I turned and spotted a little church down a side road and decided to explore. The service had already started otherwise I might have gone in. Beyond the church there seemed to be an open space, a grassed area with asphalt footpaths where people could exercise their dogs. I walked on. Eventually I came to a river. This had to be the River Spen. It was not yet ten o'clock, but all along the bank men were sitting with their fishing rods. I walked along the bank behind them. No one seemed to have caught anything and no one spoke. Fishing is a serious business. A chap with a dog came up to speak to me and urged me to approach a young man in a green peaked cap and say that I was from Kirklees Council and would he move along!

I turned and walked back into the town where I sat for a while in the Memorial Gardens. These magnificent gardens really are a pride and joy. The early bulbs had finished, but the beds were filled with tulips and pansies in contrasting colours. In the centre of the park was a raised bed of luminescent pale blue pansies surrounding the Memorial itself.

I decided to try and get a little gift for my sister and so on my way back I went into Tesco's and found a truffle-filled egg. It wasn't much. I reappeared at the house at eleven o'clock where she was having a cup of coffee. She was better, but still not right. We sat and talked. The migraine gave me the opportunity to show her some tenderness. She is otherwise apt to recoil from affection and it has to be offered subtly.

We had planned to go to a pub for lunch, where for two pounds ninety-five they do a quite outstanding Sunday lunch. Where else in 1993 can you get a roast lunch at that price? There was beef, lamb or pork, chicken pie or a vegetable medley. We both had beef with

Yorkshire pudding, roast and boiled potatoes, carrots, spring greens and peas, followed by trifle. It was excellent.

After lunch we drove back towards Halifax to Shibden Hall. This half-timbered farmhouse was built in 1420 in Schepdene (the valley of sheep) by William Otes. However, the house reflects the tastes of a much later owner, Ann Lister, who inherited the Hall in 1826. She decided to change it into a baronial hall and by her death in 1840 she had gutted the interior, demolished certain wings and replaced them in the Gothic style of the Romantics.

We walked first through the grounds down to the boating lake and sat in the sun before climbing back up to the house. We went inside, starting with the kitchen and saw the study, the parlour, the dining room and the housebody which is like a central hall with a banqueting table. The walls were all oak-clad which made it appear dark. Upstairs we saw the bedrooms and the nursery. Behind the house is a museum with horse-drawn carriages and accessories, the brewhouse. dairy and different workshops: clogger, saddler, chemist, blacksmith, wheelwright, cooper, potter and basket-maker. Among the carriages was a magnificent nineteenth century hearse. Painted black, it had an elaborate cast-iron cornice, plate glass side windows etched with floral patterns and silver-plated fittings. Inside it was draped in purple velvet. What a way to go! I could have spent hours there, but Eleanor had schoolwork to do and so we went back. I sat in the sun and read, and then mowed the grass for her.

I slept well that night and Eleanor brought me a cup of tea just after half past seven. As I was sitting there drinking it I thought to myself that I didn't remember taking my tablets. After four months it becomes an automatic action which one scarcely registers. I convinced myself that I had forgotten and took two more. Eleanor left at five past eight and I got up to have my breakfast. By nine o'clock I knew I hadn't forgotten my tablets and felt quite peculiar.

It had been my plan that morning to walk down to the town and have a cup of coffee and a bun in Watsons coffee shop, a local institution, and then to take the bus back to Dewsbury. But it was pouring with rain and I decided to take a taxi. The cat came in looking like a drowned rat. He wanted stroking and then settled down between the lounge, dining-room and kitchen doors so that I had to stop over him constantly if I wanted to move about. I sat down with a coffee and tried to read my book, but I couldn't really see the page properly.

The taxi came at twenty past twelve and in ten minutes we were in Dewsbury. I was on the coach at ten to one and tucking into my soup and sandwiches.

I had left my car in Eva's drive when I went away. On my return I discovered a carrier bag attached to the handle of the driver's door. It was rather exciting. Inside I found a bar of chocolate and a very beautiful spray of flowers which Eva had obviously picked from her garden. There were yellow roses and white·and red rhododendrons, wallflowers, lilac and cornflowers. You can imagine the scent. This gift gave me more pleasure than I can describe. It was unexpected, it was beautiful.

It was a good weekend and it took me out of myself. My sister and I had got on well together. She had been welcoming and was, I'm sure, pleased to see me. In fact, my illness seemed to have started to mend something which had gone wrong between us when our father had died. She was kinder to me, more tolerant and less sharp. I was looking forward to visiting her again.

Back in my flat I felt lonely and isolated. I felt my life had no purpose and I started thinking that maybe I should go back to work, but I knew it was more sensible to wait until September, when I would be stronger, rather than to try to slot back in at the end of the school year. The question was how I should spend the next three months. I could go to Germany or down to the South coast or even visit my friend in Philadelphia. I would have to see.

Always analytic and introspective, I was struggling desperately in my mind with certain things which had happened which had hurt me deeply. These were things that in normal circumstances I wouldn't have had time to dwell on. The problem was accepting people as they are, accepting that they are very often wrapped up in themselves, do not listen and are unaware of other people's needs, in this case mine. More difficult still was the knowledge that their stupidity and the thrust of what they said diminished or even crushed me. I was not prepared to condone this, but didn't know how to protect myself. These were people I loved, who loved me, but who were unaware of their own unconscious. Words spoken in anger can cut deeply, can reopen old wounds and sometimes there is no soothing balm. The wounds fester and you know that only time will heal, but I fear that I have no time and I don't want to take these open wounds with me to the grave.

Eva had reminded me of Descartes' words: 'To understand all is to forgive all', but I was angry, unwilling or unable to understand and certainly not in forgiving mode. She had often told me that I should not have expectations of people or else I would be disappointed. I could never agree with this. We have all manner of relationships, parent-child, brother-sister, friends, colleagues, lovers. Each one is unique. Part of these relationships are the expectations we attach to those we need to attach them to. It is what justifies them and I would just have to learn to live with the disappointments. I missed my father and Howard desperately.

In my anger and resentment I decided to throw out all my personal effects, letters, cards, photographs - every clue to my real identity. All that should remain of me was my writing. In this way I could determine what people should know, should remember of me. I could not bear the idea that anyone should have access to these things once I had gone, should pick through them like a voyeur, things which only had meaning for me. With tears rolling down my face remembering loves lost I threw them all away. All I have kept are the cards and letters Howard sent me. I cannot cast him out.

I contemplated suicide, not yet, but when the infections start to take charge of my body and I know that I am going to die. It would have to be something painless, something I could administer myself, an injection in my hand perhaps. Then, having said my goodbyes, I would go and see Eva and, when we had talked for a while, I would take out a syringe and inject its lethal contents. I would sit there holding her hand, waiting. She is the gentlest person I have ever met, unembittered after seventy hard years and many personal tragedies. But I knew I wasn't brave or decisive enough. I may not be a survivor, but I'm not a quitter and I feel obliged to see this through to the end. The appeal for me was that I could pre-empt the virus and cheat it of its moment of glory. I dismissed the idea from my mind, but did not rule it out absolutely. It might be nice for once in my life to do something out of character and surprise everybody.

There is a relatively new group in society which is being victimised. I mean the smokers. Non-smokers seem to imagine that they have licence to comment, criticise and complain. It clearly gives them a sense of superiority as if they held the moral highground. Certainly the ex-smokers are the worst. I resent very deeply the digs I have received constantly about my smoking, whether from my doctors, my mother or anyone else. "Are you cutting down?" Well, no I am not. It is something I enjoy, it keeps me calm in the face of my illness and anyway why should I? Anyone with two brain cells to rub together must realise that it won't be my smoking which will kill me. However, I do try to keep it in bounds, but it is difficult when I am sitting around all day with nothing to do. My dad gave up his pipe and it didn't do him any good. He would have been happier rubbing the Grand Cut between his hands and filling his pipe to the end. In any case I would rather that the fags killed me than this bloody virus.

Then there was Lesley, an ex-smoker, who, dealing as part of her brief in sex education with HIV and AIDS, but with limited medical knowledge, told me that my medication would be ineffective if I smoked. This was a thoughtless thing to say whether or not it was true. Until I started reading, I didn't know whether she was right or not. In fact I have read nothing to suggest that smoking is a contributory co-factor in any opportunistic infection or that it affects the efficacy of the medication in any way. Why do the people we love hurt us so much?

May God protect us from this ruddy paternalistic society which the do-gooders are intent on enforcing on us all. Why can't they concentrate their efforts on promoting washing powder or sanitary towels and let people live their lives the way they choose? I wish they would ban certain people instead. Why not ban swearing or coke cans, chewing gum or dog shit? It's my cigarettes which make my life just about bearable now.

However, I have half-promised myself that if a cure is found in time for me I will try to give up. If not, I have misgivings about everlasting life and heaven. I feel sure that there won't be people there with nasty habits like smoking and drinking, people who enjoy having sex. I feel sure it will just be people who go to church and visit National Trust houses and buy trinkets - mainly women. And no one would talk to me because I had AIDS. All in all hell would be a better bet for me. I think I would feel more comfortable with the people there. They'd be on my wavelength and I could smoke myself into oblivion. Perhaps I could even try opium.

I channelled some of my anger and resentment into my reading, challenging the NAM Treatment Updates to defy my intellect and intelligence.

I reached really only one conclusion. Insofar as the virus mutates and resistant strains can be detected in the body after only six months, it seemed to make sense to add a second drug at that stage to try to mop up the virus which had become resistant. The question was which? ddI appeared to be more strongly antiviral, but there seemed to be greater synergy when ddC and AZT were used together. In short trials ddC seemed to have the advantage over ddI in late-stage infection in terms of survival, but there seemed to be a significantly greater risk of pancreatitis and peripheral neuropathy from it.

It was time to be going back to the clinic. Dr Kapembwa had rung me the day before, wondering whether I would be prepared to take part in a trial, as a control. He didn't tell me any more. I was going to ask him again about ddI and ddC and I would find out whether my urine test had thrown any light on the tumour on my lung.

He told me that he had phoned my headmaster and told him that I was recovering well from a chest infection and getting stronger, but that the treatment would be protracted. Geoff just wanted to know, I think, how long I was likely to be out of action.

The clinic only opened last April and Dr Kapembwa is still setting up the support services for HIV patients. He talked to me about a new appointment which had been made in the Social Services Department. The new HIV liaison officer in Harrow had already rung me and I was waiting to hear from her again to arrange for her to come and see me. The idea was to prime the support services and register my name with them in case I became ill again and needed Meals on Wheels or a home help. He told me that there are also grants which are available to which HIV patients are entitled such as to pay for a telephone or to help with the cost of heating.

There was also a new dietician who was involving herself directly with the clinic and the needs of HIV patients. He didn't realise that I had an appointment to see Marion Creamer later that afternoon.

Then he spoke to me about the trial he wanted me to take part in, no obligation of course. The B-cells produce proteins, immunoglobulins, which attack and coat viruses and bacteria before they are engulfed by the macrophages. A technique for highlighting areas of inflammation and infection in the body is to inject patients with immunoglobulins which have been labelled with technetium to distinguish them from the immunoglobulins occurring naturally in the body. They then make their way to any area of infection and latch onto the invaders (pathogens) and can be seen on X-ray. Dr Kapembwa's special area of research is gut problems in HIV. Diarrhoea is very common among HIV patients and he was asking me to take part as a control because I do not appear to have any problems in that area. Was I willing? You bet. I would have to go to St Mary's hospital in Paddington two days running, 9th and 10th June, to have the injection and some X-rays.

My urine test hadn't revealed anything new about the shadow on the lung. My lymph nodes weren't swollen and he was pleased, particularly with my weight. He thinks that I am still improving and is waiting for me to reach a plateau and stabilise. At that point he will consider adding another anti-retroviral drug.

Anne bled me with Kathy holding my other hand. I can't believe how relaxed I've become about having my blood taken. It hardly bothers me at all. I went down to the pharmacy to fetch my tablets and then had my chest X-rayed. Before taking the X-ray back to the clinic I went to see the dietician. She noted my weight, eleven stone four and my height, six foot one, and took out a chart to show me my ideal weight range. I am still at the lower end and she thought it would be good if I could put an some more. I told her what I eat on a normal day, breakfast, lunch and tea and all the snacks in between. She seemed very pleased with my diet and endorsed my regime. She suggested that I could add a glass of orange juice to make sure I have sufficient vitamin C. Apparently it is easily destroyed in sunlight and so frozen vegetables are often better than fresh vegetables, which may have been lying around, as they are quick frozen within a couple of hours of being picked. She gave me a useful little pamphlet and we went off to fetch some Super Build Up which contains twice as many calories as the one I had been buying. There was a whole range of flavours, vanilla, orange, strawberry, banana and tropical fruits. I returned to the clinic well pleased. Marion is the only dietician I have met who, by her thorough, methodical approach, has helped me at all.

I had just started using the nebuliser when Dr Kapembwa burst in to show me my X-ray. The shadow was still there, but the white fluffy stuff seemed to be disappearing. I told him that I couldn't see much difference. It was not the right thing to say because he was quite excited.

It was gone seven o'clock, some four and a half hours later, when I left the hospital. The Arsenal versus Sheffield match was on at Wembley and the traffic was awful. I was worn out and had a headache. I hadn't had to wait long, I had just been busy, but Dr Kapembwa is rather long-winded and I had scarcely been given the opportunity to say the three little things I needed to say: that my legs ached, that I had a very itchy bum and that I had started sweating at night when I stopped the Pyrazinamide. This upset me and the next morning I was up at six thirty and crying into my glass of orange juice.

It was nearly the end of May and I knew that I must make a decision about my job. I didn't want to go back full-time as I feared that the stress could lead to an early progression in my infection, but I was also concerned that accidie could set in if I didn't have something to do. It didn't seem to be the right moment to change jobs; if I returned to my old job I knew what I was going back to. I knew my colleagues, I knew the system. It seemed that part-time might be the answer. I spoke again with the union and realised that if I took early retirement I was still entitled to do some teaching, but it had to be less than half a week or I would forfeit my pension. I thought this might suit quite well and I worked out that my pension and the money I would be earning would be enough to get by on. I wouldn't be able to save, but nor would I have to dig into my savings. I knew I wasn't going to reach retirement so I wanted the time now, time for myself and time for my illness. With this in mind I phoned the school and made an appointment to see the headmaster.

Driving slowly along Herkomer Road, finishing my cigarette, I felt like I was going to a funeral, probably my own, but I had a great welcome from the ladies in the office and Marian, the bursar. I slipped into the Examinations Office to see Sandra and then went along to Melissa, the headmaster's PA.

Geoff and I shook hands and I launched into my exposition. I apologised for looking disgustingly healthy, but told him I had been very ill. I had got over the pneumonia, but was still undergoing treatment for the mycobacterial infection and still had a shadow on my lung.

Dr Kapembwa said I was getting stronger and continuing to improve, but he had warned me to avoid stress. He thought I could try a little part-time work from September, but that with the demands of the new curriculum and testing it would be inadvisable to return full-time.

The treatment was going to be protracted and I didn't want to jeopardise the improvement I'd made by taking on too much. Indeed, I didn't know that a return to work full-time would be allowed in the foreseeable future.

What I was proposing, which I saw as benefiting both the school and myself, was that I should apply for early retirement on medical grounds with effect from 31st August and that I should be re-employed part-time from the beginning of the Autumn Term. I knew he wasn't keen on part-timers, but I had eighteen years' experience which I wanted to put at his disposal. If I were to return full-time, which I doubted whether I could manage yet, I would have to take time off in order to attend the hospital. My way the school wouldn't have to pay me for work I wasn't doing and I was better off with my pension and my part-time salary.

He liked the idea, thought it was neat. All in all he was marvellous, so welcoming and so eager to accommodate me. He saw the sense in what I was proposing and said he would submit it to the staffing committee with his backing. I felt like giving him a hug. I also felt that, if I need to, I can confide my HIV status to him. I can't wait to get back. After eighteen years I belong there and cannot turn my back on the place.

That evening I wrote Geoff a little card thanking him. This has given me a tremendous boost. If I can keep well and get back to work, even though only part-time, I feel it will give me a new lease of life.

I received an answer to one of my letters, Dr Kevin Cahill, Eva's friend who, I discovered, works for the Centre for International Health and Cooperation, wrote a quite encouraging letter. He drew attention to my weight increase from one hundred and twenty-six pounds to one hundred and fifty-four pounds and the fact that I had responded to two major challenges, PCP and atypical AFB. He concluded from this that the combination of my immunity and my medication was working well for me. He also urged me not to depend too greatly on numbers alone and said that he had half a dozen patients with CD4 levels below ten who were asymptomatic and fully functioning.

He thought that combination therapy was an idea I should pursue with my doctors, but he warned me that he had begun many of his own patients on the regimen I had mentioned and had had to back off when several developed pancreatitis and severe peripheral neuropathy.

Echoing my Uncle David's thoughts, he said he now viewed AIDS as a chronic challenge where every clinical problem is serious rather than the uniformly fatal disease he once knew.

I think that what he meant was really that, with the experience which has been gained of the disease, the knowledge for dealing effectively with the opportunistic infections has developed to enable doctors to prolong the lives of patients. Uniformly fatal it still is. If they can't save people like Arthur Ashe and Rudolf Nureyev, they can't save anyone at all.

I've spent a lot of time setting up my roof garden for the summer. I have replaced the perennial plants which died last year when the roof was resurfaced. I bought seven that I had never heard of. Then I got some bedding plants: salvias, nemesia, snapdragons, nicotiana and African marigolds. Peter is going to give me some petunias and some black pansies he has grown from seed. My blue rose came into flower a couple of weeks ago, it produced an enormous bloom, much too heavy for the stem, which was then beaten down by the rain. It is lightly fragrant, but my greatest pleasure is just to sit and look at it and marvel at the perfection of nature.

Last Friday I went for a swim, I've always loved swimming, I love the way the water supports your body and you feel almost weight-less. I used to go to the pool regularly and swim twenty or thirty lengths. I thought I would not try to do more than ten. The water felt cold, but I got into my stride. By the third length I was aching across and down both arms, but I was breathing all right. After five I stopped. I felt dreadful and my heart was pounding away. I had a rest. I was at the wrong end of the pool to get out so I thought I would just swim back and call it a day, but as I launched myself into my final length I started thinking to myself: 'I paid two pounds thirty for this,' so I did five more. They were a little easier. I didn't enjoy it, but I was glad I had gone. I went again on Monday. I did five lengths, had a rest and then another five. I found it much easier and enjoyed it more.

Most of all I appreciate the ordinary things in life like a swim, a drink with Julian, a chat with Lesley, walking the dog with Peter, things I have done countless times before.

There are comparatively few men in my life, just Julian, Peter, Mike and Mike and Dr Kapembwa, whom I see on a regular basis and I value their company. I marvel constantly at how so many women seem to fill their heads with the paraphernalia of life and talk unstoppably about themselves and their trifling concerns. I used to think it was a kind of defence mechanism because it effectively bars any communication from taking place, but I think now that it is rather a desire to be perceived, to be appreciated, that they are asserting that they exist and attempting to validate their existence. When St Paul bade women cover their heads he meant, so I am told, cover their whole heads – to stop them talking.

In my mind I can't equate my illness with anything I did. I suppose that's because it's so long ago. Although it seems like an act of God I know it isn't and I take full responsibility. Nothing that I think or feel can change anything, but knowing that we can experience nothing but the present moment is a comfort. Until I saw Geoff I felt like I was in no man's land, neither properly alive anymore nor actually dead yet. The prospect of returning to work is an affirmation of life. With my current medication and treatment I am starting to feel invulnerable. I just hope that I can hang on for a couple of years as there are so many new drugs being developed.

Reading back through what I have written this time I realise how very thin-skinned I have become, how easily hurt and sensitive I am. I know that no one is intentionally hurting me, it is just that I am so vulnerable.

Part Seven

I spent the Bank Holiday weekend with my mother at the house. I was still feeling apprehensive and rather wary after our row, but I had a nice time. As I parked the car Tiger trotted up to greet me as if she had been sitting waiting for me for the past three weeks. Little did she suspect that I know that she had transferred her affections to the decorator during my absence.

We went up to Polesden Lacey to see the gardens. The plants had come on a lot. The ornamental cabbages, which always make me laugh, were in full bloom as were the shrub roses. I had wanted to see the peonies, but we were too early and there were only one or two which had opened. Along the walls the clematis, acacia and wisteria made a marvellous display. We sat for a long time in the sun.

On the Saturday we walked down to the village in the morning. We were early, but it was hot like a summer's day. We stopped to talk to different women that my mother knows either from church or from when she taught or from just having lived there so long. This is what being part of a community is. I have never really experienced it apart from in the school, but there no one has time to talk.

In the afternoon we drove into Leatherhead and looked round the shops. She bought some sweets and I got a CD of Handel's Water Music.

On Sunday we went to visit my aunt in Dulwich. She is my mother's elder sister. She is eighty-two, but still plays golf regularly and enjoys a rubber of bridge. She is rather smarter than the rest of us. She didn't have children, but had a quite prestigious job in local government. She is very different from my mother and I am aware of a great difference between them which I suspect goes back to childhood.

We were joined by my other aunt, who lives in Islington. At eighty-three she is the eldest in our party. She isn't really a relative but a childhood friend of my mother and aunt from when they lived in Aberystwyth. Before the war they all came to London and lived together in a flat. I'm sure they had great fun. They still treat my mother like a younger sister. Their men have all died and they are together again.

Lunch with them is a boozy affair. They sit and drink and reminisce, I think they had a wonderful war. My aunt starts to sneeze. This indicates that the drink is going to her head. It's an entertaining afternoon for me, the observer.

Every time I put my head outside the door Tiger appeared. Sometimes she came to call and a little furry face appeared at the french windows and peered in. She definitely prefers men and it became clear to me that her great yearning for affection is really a sexual display as she gives up her whole body to my caressing hands and looks me in the eyes as if she wanted us to kiss and become one. That is our secret and I hold it locked in my heart, I'm in love with her and her dumpy sensuality.

On the Saturday night I dreamed about her. She had gone away to hide in the back garden because she had done something she was ashamed of and I was looking for her and calling: "It doesn't matter, Tiger, it doesn't matter." I wish I could love people as much as I love Tiger and forgive them as easily. I think perhaps I have forgiven myself. That is probably a good start.

On the Monday morning my mother went down to the shops to get some things and I sat in an armchair musing. I don't remember what gave rise to it, but I decided I wanted to write a book, 'Underpants through the Ages'. The more I thought about it the better the idea seemed. It would need a lot of research, but I could picture it in my mind. Egyptians, Greeks, Romans, mediaeval man all in their smalls. I wasn't sure that they had worn any. If not I would have to start from a later date with the introduction, invention or discovery of the underpants. There would have to be lots of photographs of the different garments and occasional plates with someone modelling them. The underlying sexual theme appealed to me and I felt sure that the implicit sexual content would make it a best-seller. It would be easier if I knew more about history, and, indeed, underpants.

I started having sex when I was very young, still a child. The sexual drive in me was immensely powerful. For years it dictated how I spent my time. I wasn't looking for a relationship just constantly new experiences. It was like a hobby to be pursued whenever an occasion presented itself. I never spoke to anyone about my adventures, but the desire for sex took possession of me and was too powerful to be repressed. I enjoyed these experiences with a voracity I can now hardly comprehend.

This lasted until I started work. Then I no longer had the time to pursue my hobby and the sheer dreariness of the teaching stifled my interest and reduced my appetite. I also started to change and it was no longer so clear to me what I wanted. For the last ten years I have sought sexual gratification rather half-heartedly. I needed the release, the contact of flesh on flesh, the physical catharsis, but was becoming increasingly indifferent. It may have been the action of the virus in me. It may have been my increasing awareness and unconscious fear of AIDS. I was never quite sure, and I am still not, what is safe and what is not. I know that anal sex is high risk, but I have never enjoyed that, which is why I didn't think I had put myself at risk.

I haven't had sex now since November or October or whenever the last time was. Initially when I became ill there was no response. Even now my libido is very weak. I like the idea of having sex again and once or twice a week I can perhaps tease myself into life so that I have some pleasure. I think maybe that the powerful antibiotics are repressing my libido. I am still not looking for a relationship. I have good friends who fulfil most of my needs. What I want is just good sex, but I shall have to wait a while. At least there will be no fear of getting AIDS anymore and I can make certain that I don't pass on the virus.

I am unbearably sensitised and vulnerable. It will be good when I go back to work and I have to focus on my job rather than on myself. I need to be treated very gently, but only Julian and Eva seem to be remotely aware of this. At the same time Julian doesn't really treat me any differently from before. I enjoy our wide-ranging conversations and he doesn't treat me like an invalid. How difficult other people are finding it to deal with my illness. For Julian's birthday I bought him a very beautiful little statue from the British Museum. It is a sixth century BC Greek bronze, a leaping dolphin.

I am afraid of making wrong decisions, I never worried before, but it seems so crucial now that I make the right choices. It is as though my life depends on it.

Last week Eleanor, who was on half-term, came down to London for a day. We all met up for lunch at the Kingsley Hotel, where we always go, but I was still bitterly upset and smarting from something that had happened the evening before. I'd been round to see a friend. She had been in an aggressive argumentative mood and reminded me that I had the virus for life. I went home and cried and was angry that I had once again allowed her to get under my skin and destroy a part of me I need for my fight. And yet she is kind, well-meaning and concerned, but the hurt was deep. I couldn't enjoy my food at all. How were we going to spend the afternoon? A trip on the river, a sightseeing bus? We couldn't decide. After the meal I went upstairs to the toilet. The food and alcohol and my hurt were making me tired and I leaned heavily on the top of the urinal. It was a sticky day and outside I felt sweaty and ill at ease. The noise of the buses and taxis as they rushed past was deafening, I felt I couldn't bear the noise, the people, the humidity and decided to go back home, saying I felt tired. I kissed them both goodbye and crossed the road. Five minutes later I knew it had been the wrong decision. I didn't see Eleanor often. Where had they said they were going? Dillons? I could catch up with them and at least have a cup of tea before going back. I struggled down Charing Cross Road sweating and found the shop in Trafalgar Square. There was no sign of them. It was like looking for a needle in a haystack and I decided to give up and make my way back. I stopped at a little café at the top of Shaftesbury Avenue and sat at a table outside having a cup of tea. I knew I had to get back. The tears were welling up behind my eyes.

My father's death had been a great blow to us all; he was a gentle, kind and loving man. My mother had lost a husband, lover and companion and my sister and I had lost a father, comforter and friend. Since his death we have gone away three times together. We've been to Yugoslavia and Malta and last year we went to Madeira. These holidays have not worked for me. First of all, three is not a good number. One person feels left out and that is always me. In addition, I feel uncomfortable with the unconscious expectations they have of me. They seem to project out to me what they miss in him and I am no longer brother and son, but substituting for my father, in various ways. What gets overlooked is that I miss my father too.

I remember in Dubrovnik, the first year, sitting down one evening while my mother and sister had gone to see Hamlet performed by the English National Theatre, who had come over for the festival, and spending three hours writing a letter to Howard in which I attempted to sort out what was going on between the three of us and why I was feeling so unhappy. Each time when I come back I suffer a massive reaction until I throw myself into something new, usually decorating the flat. Each time I vow I will never go again, but in the end I can never manage to say no. Eleanor wants a holiday, but won't go unless I go. It feels desperately unfair. If I say I am not keen or that I have other plans, she gets into a mood and so I relent. What will she do when I am no longer around? I am not good company when we are away; I am gruff and short-tempered. Then I feel guilty that I am spoiling their holiday.

My sister is like a little girl in her excitement before we go and quite relentless in her determination to see and do everything while we are away. Sometimes she looks at me in a way I don't recognise or understand and can't interpret or respond to. It is as though she has gone away with her parents long ago before I came on the scene and spoiled everything for her. I wish these holidays worked for me, but I can't pretend they do. Moreover, they seem to be damaging to my relationship with both my mother and my sister. I wish they would go away on their own and not insist that I come too, I know they would have much more fun.

Anyway I've agreed again. She caught me off-guard with a phone call last Saturday morning. Would I like to go to Switzerland? I had already said quite firmly that I would not consider any of the southern countries. It sounded like a nice idea when she suggested it and, in a moment of weakness, I agreed, but I can't see how it can be any better than before. Nothing has really changed.

Yugoslavia, Malta and Madeira were in other respects marvellous holidays. Dubrovnik, pearl of the Adriatic, is superb. Malta is steeped in history and I have never seen anywhere more beautiful than Madeira. I loved the rugged North coast with its areas of rain forest, the flowers everywhere on the island growing wild, I took hundreds of photographs each time.

We were rather late booking and couldn't find anywhere suitable in Switzerland so we are off to the Grand Bristol Hotel on Lake Maggiore in northern Italy. I know it is going to be too grand for me. It's certainly far too expensive. Eva has been to the lake and tells me it is absolutely heaving with people and cars in the summer, it sounds like the sort of place I will hate. At least it has brought my mother and me closer together. She enjoys the holidays more than I do, but doesn't really want to go either. We console one another. I hope so much that the holiday may turn out to be a right decision, but that does not lie only in my hands. I do wish we were going to the seaside, but there is really no point because I can't risk swimming in the Med.

Lesley had offered me a lift to St Mary's, but I had declined, explaining that this was a little adventure for me and that it was not so adventuresome if I was delivered to the front by car.

I had parked the car in what seemed like the last space available and was waiting to cross the Kenton Road when a black Porsche drew up and an Asian chap asked me the way to Northwick Park, I pointed out the road and said I was also going there. I crossed the road and he turned the car round on the crossing and then he pulled up again. I got in and off we sped. He smelled good, freshly showered. I complimented him on his car. We drove round and round looking for a space. In the end he dropped me at the station and carried on looking by himself.

I feel comfortable with the ethnic minorities, perhaps because I belong to a minority group myself. The only difference is that I can conceal it and they of course can't and have to live with people's prejudices. A lot of the English I find physically unattractive and really rather arrogant. I'm sure it is a leftover from when we had an empire of subjugated peoples. There is nothing like asserting one's authority over someone else in order to feel superior. Unfortunately this seems to have become a national characteristic with too many English people regarding foreigners as inferior. The fact that we had been on the winning side in both wars hadn't contributed to our humility either. I believe it is possible to talk in terms of national characteristics and some of the less attractive ones I would associate with the English are that they are very often ignorant, intolerant and prejudiced. I am no doubt bitter because I have been on the receiving end of their prejudices expressed through the mouthpiece of their children. As a teacher living and working in Germany I was not made to suffer in this way but was welcomed as a guest in their country.

It is eleven o'clock and I am sitting here waiting in the Department of Clinical Physics on the third floor of the Queen Elizabeth the Queen Mother wing (known as the QEQM to the initiated) in St Mary's. It is very swish. You should have seen the control panels in the lift (it had two). There are strange scientific noises behind the scenes as things are raised and lowered hydraulically. There are monitors and strange machines and men in white coats. There is a big tank with some fish and some pieces of weed, I think, which also seem to be swimming around purposefully. I am very excited. Ken Wise, Senior Medical Technician, comes and calls my name. He looks irritated as I insist on finishing my sentence, but I have had to wait twenty-five minutes.

The injection only took a moment and I was put to sit with the fish for ten minutes. Then they started to take pictures of me, chest and abdomen, two from above and two from below. Each one took five minutes and I had to lie still. My face immediately started to itch.

I was to report back at four o'clock for more pictures. I had a lunch at Garfunkel's, breast of chicken with mushrooms in a cheese sauce. It was delicious, but much too much for me. I walked along to the Edgware Road and had a look round the shops, but it was drizzling and I didn't have my umbrella. I made my way back to a little patisserie across the road from the hospital and sat myself down at the back with a pot of tea.

Several men with stethoscopes slung nonchalantly round their necks and pagers on their belts came in and bought themselves pieces of cake. And then in walked Professor Pasvol. I went up to him and invited him to join me for a cup of tea. He couldn't, he had a meeting and was already late. I wasn't bothered because I was trying to get into conversation with a very pretty girl who had chosen to sit down at the table next to mine and asked to share my ashtray. She was wearing scarlet leggings and a T-shirt. French, I thought. But for the fact that she smoked I wouldn't have spoken to her. She was Italian, from Sicily, and was in London for the summer doing a language course. I told her I was going to Lake Maggiore in the summer and made some comment about the Sicilian Mafiosi. She told me that the Mafia were throughout Italy, not only in Sicily, and many politicians were involved. If you spoke out publicly against them you had to watch your back. She complained that there wasn't much going on in Sicily. If you wanted to open a disco or a business you had to pay protection money. Her English was quite adequate, in fact she had a very wide vocabulary. It was an interesting way of passing the time until four o'clock. I think she had welcomed our conversation as much as I had.

They wanted me back at nine o'clock the next morning. This was a tall order. I had to take my tablets at timed intervals before breakfast and then there were my bowels. I got up at six o'clock and was on my way at twenty-five past seven. I got to Paddington in record time and at ten past eight I was back in Garfunkel's having a cup of coffee. I didn't have to wait at all in the hospital, but was taken straight in by Ken Wise. He is a diffident, somewhat troubled young man and stood talking to me for a lot of the time while the pictures were being taken. This relieved the monotony as each one took twenty minutes. He explained to me what they were doing. Since the injection the previous day I had been radioactive. These were gamma rays, not X-rays. The pictures that morning were taking longer as the radioactivity had been disintegrating in my body overnight. The machine contained a crystal which detects radioactivity and after intensification the findings are converted into images for the computer. By injecting me with antibodies they were able to detect the presence of any pathogens in my body. The process was still in an experimental stage, but it was hoped that one day it would enable them to target treatment so precisely that it would lead to the elimination of cancer and other infections.

The image showed clearly my heart, liver, kidneys and bladder, areas of high blood penetration. I feel very pleased that I have been involved in this. I feel I have contributed something to medical science.

The Wellcome conference has been taking place in Berlin this week and I heard on the radio that companies are now producing AIDS self-testing kits which detect the presence of antibodies in the saliva. These are illegal in this country. What would you do if you found you were positive, go to the chemists and get some aspirin? I was interested to hear that they are still estimating thirty million cases of HIV world-wide by the year 2000. Will I be one of them or will I be long gone? I was reminded of my anger when Howard tested positive. Some people fuck and fuck and get a baby, others get AIDS. Perhaps chemists should produce combination packs of pregnancy and AIDS self-testing kits. There is no justice, no fairness.

Dr Robert Gallo, to whom I had written and from whom I had received no response, was speaking at the conference. An accidental observation had revealed that a harmless virus carried by most of the population could be used to block infection of the white blood cells by the AIDS virus. The virus, a member of the herpes family, locks onto the same receptor sites as HIV. Laboratory tests show that the Human Herpes Virus-7 (HHV7) can prevent HIV infection in cell cultures. This has opened up a new attack against HIV. They are to identify the protein surrounding the virus which enables it to lock onto the white blood cells. It may then be possible to deliver this protein to patients to block the receptor site on the cell.

One other piece of news which may be important is that powerful new drugs for treating flu may soon be available. Using computer-aided biochemical techniques to build a model of the structure, they have designed two compounds that inhibit the growth of the flu virus. It is hoped that this technology may be used in designing new anti-AIDS drugs.

I decided to go to the hospital rather earlier than usual and have my lunch in the restaurant so that I would have a break from cooking. I set off at about half past twelve and had a filling, if not particularly good, lunch. I made my way to the dietician's office and sat and waited for her. As I sat there I started to feel sad, incredibly sad, I could feel the tears building up behind my eyes. I saw Marion and then went to the clinic. I was pleased with my weight at nearly eleven and a half stone. Dr Kapembwa shook my hand and, looking at me, said: "You've lost your sparkle." I told him he was right, that I was feeling heavy-hearted and then the tears started. He leaned forward towards me, took my hand and told me to take my time and let it all come out. I did, but there was nothing new, just the same old things which were causing me to hurt, which I was aware of and struggling to deal with: the unconscious messages I was receiving from some of the people around me, the casual comments which diminished me, the overwhelming feeling not of loneliness but of being alone, my doubts about my writing. He told me that my tears were quite normal; as people start to get physically stronger, they can be overwhelmed by their emotional response to the infection. It was a delayed grief reaction, not uncommon in advanced HIV infection. We talked about the possibility of my seeing an HIV counsellor. I said I wanted a man. I felt surrounded by women, my mother, my sister, my doctor, my analyst, my colleagues. There was a gap in my life since my father died, which could only be filled by an older man. I wanted a wise old man, intelligent, intuitive, experienced and knowledgeable. Unfortunately, these are very thin on the ground. I suggested Solomon. I told Dr Kapembwa that he fulfilled this role for me and he invited me to ring the clinic any time I needed to talk to him. However, he felt I should see someone with more specialised knowledge of the emotional side of HIV. I think it is probably too late; I have already cast him in that role. I don't want, don't need anyone else when I have him. I shall have to make do with the half hour I spend with him once a month. He doesn't need to do anything, just be there for me while I'm with him. He is intelligent, sensitive and feeling, and I feel safe with him.

I felt I didn't understand the tears, the upsurge of grief or how it had been triggered. The meal hadn't been that bad or perhaps it had. I had chosen lamb which came in a very thick gravy with roast potatoes. I hadn't liked it much and the potatoes had tasted odd. I had sat there for twenty minutes shovelling it in, telling myself that I must try to finish it. As a child I was fortunate enough to be able to go home for lunch. On one occasion on my return to school I remember seeing a little boy sitting outside the headmistress's room with a bowl of pudding. He must have been told that he had to sit there until he finished it. I was now that little boy eating up my food.

Perhaps the tears were signalling to me my ever increasing emotional dependence on Dr Kapembwa and were an excited anticipation of seeing him again. I felt guilty that I had thought him long-winded. He took a great deal of time with me, time which I needed, time which was precious to me.

Thank goodness I had decided not to set so much store by my CD4 count; it was down to sixty-two. I told him I was off to Italy at the end of July and asked if I would need any vaccinations. He said I could have hepatitis A on the spot. He told me I didn't have any antibodies to hepatitis B in my blood and suggested I might like to have a series of three injections, certainly it would be advisable if I was planning on having multiple sexual partners. As it is difficult to break the habit of a lifetime and this sounded quite an attractive proposition I decided it would be a wise precaution. I can be quite unpredictable in my sexual behaviour and it is better to be safe than sorry.

After Anne had taken my blood and given me the hepatitis A vaccine in my thigh and I had used the nebuliser, I went to see Karen, but I was feeling washed out emotionally and was wanting to go home. Strangely, the tears hadn't fully assuaged my grief.

The next day I started to understand why I had been so distressed. The day before I went to the clinic I had received a visit from the Social Services in the afternoon. The HIV liaison officer had come round bringing my Care Manager with her. He was an overweight young man with a moon-like face and two big earrings who stared at me without blinking, I swear, for an hour and a half like I was a freak. The whole time he was in my flat not a flicker of a smile or any expression crossed his face and on the few occasions that he spoke it was in a jargon which left me none the wiser. She had talked incessantly and I had found her rather insensitive. The whole visit had seemed grossly intrusive. Had they come to commiserate, to explain what services they could offer or just as voyeurs? I wasn't sure and I was angry that I had allowed myself to be drawn into all that chat, I didn't want to be reminded that one day I may become too ill to fend for myself. If that happens it will be time to throw in the towel.

I phoned her up to say that the young man wasn't suitable. I couldn't allow someone like that to have access to my life.. All I needed was a phone number I could ring if I felt I needed some assistance. I didn't want someone to keep a watchful eye on me. If this wasn't acceptable we could forget the whole business.

By contrast my visit from Janet Chater, health visitor from the chest clinic, had been a treat. It was she whom I had seen at the end of January when my chest infection was discovered. She is a big woman who likes to chat. I think it was quite a struggle for her to get up the forty-five steps to my flat and she was panting when she arrived. She walked in and slipped on the rug in the hall and fell flat on her back. I was so embarrassed for her. We had a good old chin-wag. She is without prejudice.

I phoned Vic and Edna, Howard's parents, the other night. They had sent me a couple of post-cards and I wanted to keep in touch. I spoke to Edna. She asked me how I was. I said I was all right, but she must have detected an uncertainty in my reply and asked me what was wrong. I told her. She was naturally upset for me and insisted I come round. I hadn't wanted to tell her over the phone, but I find it impossible to lie. I thought about Howard, how much braver he had been than me. He had only told two people, his brother and myself. I have told all the people I am close to and am still struggling.

I had always got on superbly well with Howard's grandmother, Mrs Willoughby, I used to tell Howard I wanted her to adopt me. I always liked to take her something when I went round and so I went to the florist to get some flowers. I found an exquisitely pretty, pale pink miniature rose.

Vic and Edna are fine people. I hadn't seen them for nearly two years, but they looked well and I had a great welcome. We sat on the patio in the shade and talked. We talked about me. They wanted to know the whole story and I was pleased to tell them. We talked about Howard. It was interesting that we had independently reached some of the same conclusions, that he had picked up the salmonella in Tunisia.

It is strange going to visit and Howard isn't there, and we sit in the garden where we had celebrated his twenty-first birthday ten years ago to the week. As we sat round the table and talked about him he was somehow with us again. We all have such fond memories of him. I wonder who will be sitting round a table remembering me and conjuring up my presence when I am gone? The difference between Howard and me is that I will come back to haunt, to collect, Howard to comfort.

I didn't see Mrs Willoughby. She was having a bad day and hadn't got up. She was entitled to stay in bed if she wishes, she is ninety-six. I was pleased to hear that Howard's brother Ian and his wife Louise had had a baby, little Eleanor.

I had a marvellous afternoon. Suddenly I had two parents again, two people who are genuinely fond of me, but are not involved in the same way as my own family. And there was actually a man present in my life for once. This felt good.

Vic used to work at British Aerospace in Hatfield before he retired and I remember being invited to an open day one summer. Howard and I spent most of the morning being silly in between watching the planes fly past. I can still see the Harrier jump-jet and hear its apocalyptic roar. Lunchtime came and the drinks seemed to be free. (Actually they weren't. Vic was paying, but Howard and I didn't realise this.) We drank a lot before we started on the wine or maybe it was champagne. The food was lavish. Important clients were being entertained. Howard and I sat there giggling. God knows how many billions of pounds worth of business we lost for British Aerospace that day. The Hatfield branch has subsequently closed down.

Then came the highlight of the day, helicopter rides at ten pounds a flight. It was Howard's birthday so I treated him. He sat in the front with the pilot. We had had so much to drink we scarcely knew which way was up as we shot into the sky and swooped and circled round. It was totally exhilarating. It was like riding round in the sky in a mini. This was one of the golden moments of my life.

I still feel if my mum hadn't broken her wrist and I had been able be with Howard that we were so close that I could perhaps have breathed new life into him.

I have been putting off now for months two things which require my urgent attention: my will and my funeral. I suppose I feel that when I have dealt with them I will have effectively wrapped up my life.

The will is the easier of the two. As I said back in December I want to remember all my friends with a small amount of money. I shall leave a tidy sum to the clinic which has cared for me and the rest I have decided to split three ways between my mum, my sister and a charity, probably Save the Children. It is more difficult to know how to divide up my possessions. If people will have pleasure from them, they are welcome to them.

The funeral is another matter. I know I must be cremated so that every last trace of the virus is destroyed, but as I sit here wondering what music I want played, that I want people to remember and associate with me, I draw a blank. Nothing I would choose is either suitable or short enough. The hymns are easier to select and I think I would like 'All things bright and beautiful' and 'Jesu, lover of my soul'.

One thing I do know for certain is that I want a poem read out. It is *Der Asra* by Heinrich Heine. Heine suffered from a progressive illness of luetic origin which is perhaps hinted at in the theme of this poem. It has always been my favourite. It combines in a unique way the two themes of sex and death, the former being the cause of and leading to the latter, the two taboo subjects which are embodied in AIDS. It is the sad tale of an Arab slave who falls in love with a Sultan's daughter. He sees her every evening at the fountain. Every day he becomes paler and paler. One evening the princess approaches him and asks him his name and his background. The slave answers. His name is Mohamet and he is from the tribe of Asra in Yemen. His people die when they fall in love. Really I would like to read it out myself so perhaps I'll tape it.

As for my ashes I am undecided. A part of me wants them to be buried in the churchyard in Fetcham where I grew up and a part of me wants them to be cast into the sea from the promenade between Felpham and Bognor where I would have so loved to have lived.

However, I do not want to create a logistical problem if there will be a resurrection by asking for half to be buried and half to be tossed into the sea. What to do?

In one respect I feel I have been undoubtedly fortunate. After I tested positive in November I was immediately admitted to hospital. Since then I have been on sick leave. I will have had nine months to come to terms with my infection before I return to work. How other people manage who have to go back the next day I cannot imagine. I have needed all the time to adjust.

Even now I am still frightened of the future and what it holds for me; I am frightened of getting ill and I am frightened of dying.

I have been at pains to try to resolve everything before I die and create harmony. I realise now that this is an impossible quest because it involves other people who do not share the same desire. This has caused me to become frustrated. All I can hope for is that I can become resolved within myself and achieve my own harmony. In my life there have been many occasions when I have been lonely. In the last analysis we are all on our own and only answerable to ourselves and (if we believe) God.

I have continued to remove the junk from my life, the physical and the mental, so that I will be able, I hope, to move on unencumbered.

The roof garden is quite beautiful this year with the roses, lupins, delphiniums and bedding plants. I've been back to Polesden Lacey to see the pergola with the tiny button-like white roses. They were delightful.

My attitude towards my infection has been changing. Having explored the different treatment options and realised that all the drugs are relatively ineffective and most quite toxic, it seems to me now that the important thing is to avoid having side-effects. I had deliberately not phoned the clinic to find out my CD4 count in May. If I looked well and felt well perhaps I was well and didn't need a number between nought and a thousand put on it.

The combination of my immunity and my medication seems to be working well for me. It seems to me that the fewer drugs I take the better. Then if I get sick I should derive the most benefit from them. The weeks pass and I feel fitter and fitter. It seems like my infection is only an illusion. Twice a week I am down at the pool swimming my twenty lengths and feeling fine.

I have felt very angry with some of the people around me. I am angry that they are finding my infection so difficult to deal with and won't talk about it and so there is no way I can help them. I feel that they are failing me and allowing their problems to get in the way. Occasions which could have been shared and enjoyable have been missed. I suppose it is how I feel about my life, a series of missed opportunities. My father used to say we all had our cross to bear.

My mother seems to have derived strength from my illness and my need to be cared for. I had seen this happen before with my father as she took control. Roles were allocated, nurse and patient. Now that I am well she is slow to adjust and insists continuing to treat me and talk about me as if I were an invalid. She must accept the fact that I am much better and allow me to be well. It will not last for ever.

I have even fallen out with Eva. I went to see her needing reassurance, but I put her under too much pressure and she became defensive and very angry with me.

I felt she was letting me down and shutting the door on me. I am just surprised that she couldn't see what I was so desperately craving. It certainly wasn't a brawl, I just want the status quo to prevail and I had felt it was under threat. This is a very great blow for me after twenty-two years. I feel I am losing my greatest ally.

I thought to myself that either she wasn't well, as had happened in the past, or else that it was something to do with my vulnerability. People just didn't seem to be able to cope with it and ended up attacking me. I felt then that I had done something wrong, that I probably deserved it. Even Eva seemed to have succumbed to this. There was I with my failing immune system and no defences. People just couldn't deal with it.

As a child I was never bullied, I just got on with my life and let others get on with theirs. Different I had always been, but now I felt my vulnerability was making me a target. It seems to be a human failing to want to dominate someone who is frail, sometimes out of excessive concern, sometimes not.

It was this vulnerability, both real and supposed, which was the stumbling block for most people. I was becoming everyone's favourite victim. Then when I stood up for myself, asserted myself, people seemed to feel threatened and didn't like me very much.

Having been for a short while dependent on them, it was as though they felt I now belonged to them and were reluctant to relinquish that hold, as if I had become an extension of themselves and was no longer an independent autonomous individual.

All I really need from people is to be there for me and love me and let me fight my battle in the only way I know without too much well-intentioned advice. A little is welcome, it shows they care. What I didn't like was the attention that this infection was bringing me. I am a quiet person and really just like to be left to get on. Conflict I cannot cope with.

I realise I have to be kinder and more tolerant of people's shortcomings and limitations if I am to enjoy the rest of my life. I must not expect so much from them; they are undoubtedly doing their best, but my needs are so very great now.

All in all it will be much easier for everyone when I am dead. Then there will be no one to ask the awkward questions or make the uncomfortable observations. People will be able to breathe a sigh of relief and get on with their preordained lives. No questions, no answers required.

Several people who have come to my flat, including the social worker and the young man with the moon-face, have been unable to accept a cup of tea prepared by my AIDS-infected hands. The finals students (I would have failed them all) could not eat a sweet which I had kept in my AIDS-infected room. These people are all frightened that I will contaminate them either with my infection or my smoke.

Sometimes I feel I have achieved nothing in my life. I haven't married, I don't have children, I don't have a lover. I'm not even very good at my job. I haven't produced anything worthwhile, anything by which I might be remembered. When I die it will be as though I had never lived. I have no more significance than the little wood-louse who trundles along outside, probably less. He has babies who will mourn his passing. If there is no resurrection for him then, as sure as hell, there will be none for me.

I received an answer to another of my letters, Dr Linda Distlerath from Merck Pharmaceutical Company sent me a tremendously comprehensive review on Preventive Health Care for Adults with HIV Infection. Her letter was also informative and her offer of further assistance kind. I am grateful to her for having taken the trouble to reply.

I haven't heard anything from my other three letters. They probably think they are too grand to write back to me. In a way I feel I have laid myself open, exposed myself, but I am nonetheless glad I wrote. It serves as a reminder to the researchers that there are individuals, real people, like myself whose future lies in their hands, it underscores the urgency of their work.

I still wish sometimes that I had died rather than having to continue knowing I will never be properly well again, and that my continuing good health lies in the hands of others. I don't want this kind of dependence on anyone whoever they are and however kind.

This is a story without a happy ending, but perhaps there can be some happiness, some joy, some new experiences on the way. I can see how much I have grown in the last seven months through my tears and my fears. If we can admit our frailties to ourselves then we can grow.

I realise that what I have been writing about is life and living and how very much alive I am. I am perhaps more alive than I have ever been. It is since, for the first time in my life, I felt the closeness of death and the reality of dying. I am conscious of being as never before.

Part Eight

There are certain inexplicable signs in nature, mysteries which will never be unravelled. One of these for me has been the appearance of herons at significant times in my life.

It was shortly after my father's death when I was visiting my mother, who was still very distraught, that we went to Claremont Gardens, outside Esher, for a walk one afternoon. It was a grey day and drizzling on and off. It was a perfect reflection of our mood. We wandered round and then came down to the lake. Standing on the edge in the shallow water was a grey heron, like a statue, a symbol. We sat on a bench and watched him for ages, not speaking. He moved slowly, deliberately, pausing for long periods. He stayed there with us until we had to go home.

The afternoon that I learned of Howard's death I took the car and drove out to the woods near Chessington, walked through the trees and the undergrowth remembering the friend I loved, the young man with the open, friendly face who had been so full of life and love and fun. I came to a couple of ponds and on the far side, immobile, were two herons. I tried to approach them, but the path led into the pond. I made my way back. They were still there and I could see them standing majestically in the water.

Two years ago when I was spending a few days on the South coast in Felpham I went for a walk along the prom one evening. The sun was low in the sky but still shining and the tide was miles out in the bay leaving a great expanse of sand uncovered. There on the edge, delicately dipping their feet, were three herons. Ever since that evening I had feared that I had this infection and that the third heron 'had come to call me to join my father and Howard. These are the only three occasions I have ever seen a heron. They are magnificent birds, stately and reptilian. It seems to me that they are the counterpart of the stork who delivers new life; they appear when our time is up.

I had undoubtedly been enjoying my time off work. In some respects I felt happier than I had been in years. At last I had the time to pursue my own interests and to go out and enjoy myself. This was a change from sitting at home night after night and at weekends preparing lessons that no one was interested in; marking, writing assessments and reports or entering pupils for examination on the computer and sorting out administrative problems. I was thinking also how, in two months' time, I would be back at that school and how even part-time work in teaching does not allow you much time for yourself. I wasn't sure that the decision to return to work was well-founded. Did I really want to go back and face the constant aggravation and abuse or was I just trying to prove to myself that I could still do it?

I needed a new medical certificate and went back to see Dr Segal. She said that I looked better than she had ever seen me look. All the stress had disappeared from my face.

In the evening Peter came round. It was his birthday and we had a few glasses of wine. During the night I woke up at half past one to go to the toilet and then I had a glass of orange juice and a cigarette, I knew that, if I went back to work, I would only be marginally better off. It was time to do some calculations. These seemed to show that any financial benefit to me would be minimal. I had said I would never go back. I had paid my contributions for eighteen years. Perhaps now really was the time to give up.

The next morning I woke up with an erection, the first early morning erection in what seemed like ages. No ordinary erection this, it was rock hard, enormous. I was absolutely priapic, I felt terrific. If I didn't go back to work I could do voluntary work in the clinic. Karen could use me for her condom demonstrations if she had any big enough!

Then I remembered two thoroughly unpleasant year eleven students I had taught. Theirs had been the love match of the year. They used to sit at the back of my classroom holding hands. On one occasion it had been pretty obvious that it was no longer hands which were being held under the desk and I asked the boy to move to the front. With great reluctance, not surprisingly, he complied and then, in defiance, proceeded to eat a Mars bar in my lesson. I asked him to leave the room. I was livid. I flung the door open and he thrust his desk forward with his feet and it caught my hand against the open door. The whole class realised it might be broken. In fact, we three got on very well together after this. I am not so old that I don't remember sitting in the back row of the cinema myself.

Their relationship didn't last the year. He bestowed his favours on someone new. There was a big fight between the two girls and the original girlfriend was ostracised by the whole year group. They had been envious of her courage in having a sexual relationship with the boy she loved and were relieved she had had her comeuppance. I felt sorry for her. She was a pretty girl and deserved better treatment. He was the only pupil I ever taught who failed his GCSE outright. After nearly three years he knew almost nothing at all, I think he only wrote half a line in the exam. It didn't bother me, he obviously had other qualities and attractions which would stand him in better stead in life than GCSE German. He would make out.

As I hadn't heard anything from the school I decided to ring and find out whether I had been timetabled for any lessons in September. I spoke to Bob. I was down for twelve. This sounded all right to me until I decided to work out exactly how much money I'd be getting; it was fifteen hundred pounds less than my invalidity benefit, which I would lose the moment I went back to work. I was entitled to do about twenty lessons a week without forfeiting my pension, even that only exceeded my benefit by three hundred a year after I had deducted tax and National Insurance. This seemed absurd, I was caught in a trap, I wanted to work, but if I did there was no financial benefit for me. In fact I would be worse off.

Clearly I had a choice, either to return or not. Unconsciously the choice was already made as I planned to contact the school again so that they could advertise for a replacement for me. There was no incentive to go back unless just to occupy myself. I knew all about the stress involved in teaching; there must surely be more enjoyable ways of spending one's time. However, I had been at that school for eighteen years, nearly half my lifetime. It had been rough and tough, but there had been good times in the past. The letting go was going to be more difficult than I would have imagined. I didn't feel a sense of relief or release at the prospect of giving up this job I claimed to hate, I felt rather weighed down by a great uneasiness and concern. It seemed like it was that job or nothing. What could I possibly do if I didn't go back? If I returned to work I avoided this question. It would take courage not to return, I felt sure it would hasten my death if I didn't have a real purpose and I felt I was bound to make the wrong decision whatever I did. There was also a measure of guilt. Why should I be able to give up work when other people I knew didn't have the same opportunity? It was now that I missed Eva as I turned all these things over in my mind.

That afternoon I went down to the pool. It was very empty, which I like, and I started ploughing up and down in the section reserved for lane swimming. Some minutes later a family appeared, grandparents, daughter and grandson. The boy, who was about ten, jumped in and started swimming lengths. He didn't go fast, but he was very determined. His mother didn't get in at first, but walked slowly up and down beside him on the edge. He impressed me and I resolved that, when I had finished my swim, I would tell him what a good swimmer I thought he was. I stopped at one end with his grandparents, as I thought, and spoke to his grandmother about him. In fact she was his aunt. The woman and her son were over from Poland. She lamented to me how anxious his mother was and added that that was the problem when there was no father around. The boy drew level with us and stopped. I turned to him and conveyed in sign language and very clear English how well I thought he swam. He beamed all over his face and carefully said: "Thank-you." When I left the pool, I waved goodbye to him. A little wave and again that smile, a smile that touched my heart. It had all been so simple and I felt there had been more reward for me that afternoon than in all those years teaching. This incident was a turning point for me. There might be different ways in which I could make a contribution, it would all be so much easier if I had a partner and didn't feel so alone. Friends and family just didn't seem to be enough any more.

When I told Julian of my decision he seemed at first not to approve and reminded me that I needed a purpose, but he is financially quite astute and soon grasped the true nature of the problem. I think he is perhaps a little envious, but then he is losing sight of what I have to come to terms with and face up to. I don't think anyone would really want to be in my position.

Three days later, the last day of the summer term, I braced myself and rang the school again. I spoke to Geoff. I explained my dilemma and told him I couldn't afford to come back in September. He seemed to think it was better for me to wait until I was fully fit before returning. Little did he know.

As I won't be going back at the beginning of the Autumn term I have changed the date on my early retirement form from the end of August to the end of November, when my hundred days on half pay run out. It will ensure that I have a little more money coming in. Then the school will want a clarification regarding my position and intention. Will I be coming back or not? That gives me four more months to think about what I am going to do, explore a few options and discover whether I think my life can be fulfilling without a regular job. The financial aspect doesn't have a part to play; there is no way I can improve my position, unless I give up the pension and go back full-time.

What I really want to do is to return to work, forget about the last year and pretend that none of it happened, that it wasn't real, but I know it's not a dream and I know there will be no awakening and I know there is no escape.

I have sorted out my differences with Eva and have gone back to her. She says that she thinks we will last approximately the same length of time. I find this a comfort. I have felt there were occasions when she wasn't quite tuned into me, but I am very glad to be seeing her again. I cannot afford to put away from me the people I love and who love me. She is a wise old bird and will stick by me and advise me to the end. If she can't perceive me, and relate to me then no one can.

Before my holiday I went one more time to the clinic. Dr Kapembwa still thinks I'm experiencing a delayed grief reaction. I'm not sure. He didn't know me before I got sick. I've always found life quite difficult. He had been able to think of one trained psychologist who has experience with HIV patients, but he is younger than I am. That's no good for me, I need someone older, perhaps a lot older, someone with more experience of life than me not less. And in any case it is not so critical now that I have got Eva back. He examined me and discovered that the thrush had returned. He prescribed a course of tablets for five days. He seemed pleased with me and said that my parameters were still rising. This sounded hopeful whatever it actually meant.

I told him that I wanted the series of hepatitis B injections and then we talked about my holiday. I am to have a vaccination against typhoid, just in case. Salmonella seems to be the main danger and I am to drink bottled water. I am not to eat sandwiches unless they are freshly prepared in front of me. He suggested I could make my own using tinned meat or fish. Hot meals must also be fresh and cooked the same day and I mustn't have food which has been reheated. He stressed the need for normal hygiene, washing hands in soap and water after using the toilet and before eating. He also gave me a course of antibiotics which I am to take if I get a bout of diarrhoea while I'm away. Then he said he was going to make me dynamic. I just laughed; he stands more chance of curing the HIV.

The thrush was a bit of a blow. It was very mild and I couldn't even see it myself though I could feel a little toughness at the back of my throat with my tongue, it cleared up after one tablet, but it was a reminder that the virus is still there working away at undermining my defences. The scan that was done at St Mary's hadn't shown up any infection.

The clinic was very busy that afternoon and I had to wait around for long periods and take my turn. I asked Dr Kapembwa how many HIV patients he had in the clinic. He said there were forty and that he was considering opening a second clinic. I had asked this question some months before. I think it was Kathy who told me there were about twenty. Heaven help us if this is a national trend.

I feel like I'm in partnership with Dr Kapembwa and that we will face any problems together. This makes it all feel less daunting for me, but it must be very demanding for him. He has forty other people who have the same needs as me and everyone likes to feel special. I think he likes me. When I die a little part of him will die too.

The vaccinations were intramuscular and I had one in each thigh. Ade gave me them. The typhoid was a tiny needle and I didn't feel a thing, but the hepatitis B was enormous, like an elephant's tusk and it felt like it as I clutched desperately onto Anne's hand and wound my feet six times round the base of the stool. Strangely it was the typhoid which hurt far more the following day.

The infection has raised other issues for me again, primarily my homosexuality. It was never something I had a choice about, I seemed to have been born like this; I never wanted to be different. I can identify factors in my upbringing and relationships which might seem to support the view that it is a developmental or experimental problem, but I don't really think so. Not even my analysis has been able to make a difference, to uncover any measure of heterosexuality. I like women well enough and generally get on with them well, but they do not excite me. My homosexuality is as wholly natural to me as heterosexuality is to most people.

Apart from the prejudice which exists, and which I became aware of for the first time when I started work, I enjoy having sex and am comfortable with my sexuality. Why do people have to abuse other people who are in some way different from them? The shouts of Paki, Jew-boy, woofter are demeaning, diminishing and they hurt I know; I've been the target.

When I was in my mid-twenties I decided it was time to tell my parents and my sister. It was a strange experience; I felt I was talking about someone else, someone I had made up. I think they would have rather not known and it certainly didn't help me. It was my secret and I had given it away. I swear I never functioned so well again after that.

It is terribly important to do the conventional things in life, get married, have children, watch over them as they grow up and find their way. The family line continues, the genes are propagated and death is not so final. For some of us, however, for whatever reason, this is not an option, and we are excluded from the pleasures which normal family life affords. We cannot conform and we have to discover our own way, forge a unique path. It takes courage which we don't all have or at least not all the time. Our attempt may fail, certainly it is set about by hazards. It is not an option a wise man would choose.

I have heard back from the publishers (I wrote to four) who all seem interested in what I've written. If it can be published I will feel that these months of convalescence won't have been wasted. I will have told my story and it will be on record that I existed. It should make it easier for me to die. I will be able to let go knowing that I am leaving something of myself behind. I will still be here in my writing. It is in a very real sense my child and, like a parent I feel protective towards it, jealous of it.

I should have been over the moon; it is no mean achievement to turn an AIDS infection to account, but I just felt rather flat and a bit depressed. I have so many misgivings about what I've written and have felt inclined to scrap large sections. Have I imagined or made up some of the things I've said? Will it cause offence to people I love? Is it a product of AIDS dementia? Is it just plain boring? However, when I think back I can still recall the thoughts, the feelings, the sadness which have found expression here.

I hope that what I've written may strike a chord with some people and may open the way to some discussion and an exchange of thoughts and feelings which may be enriching. Every time I tell my story I feel a little of the burden is lifted. By sharing it with people I indulge their sympathy and feel less alone. By publishing it I am offering it to the world. People may think what they like, I am not ashamed. This infection is a high price to pay for being different, for making what may have been a single mistake. It's a harsh world where a man can't afford to make a couple of little mistakes.

I've been getting myself ready for the holiday. I've bought a very grim sweatshirt in battleship grey. It needs something to liven it up like a gold brooch or sequins! I also got a very jolly pair of patchwork shorts in blue, green, red and purple. Then I treated myself to two short-sleeved silk shirts which were reduced in the sale. One is mulberry (again) and the other is mid-blue. They are the sort of colours which just scream out: 'This shirt is silk'. I've never had silk before, but I was worried I'd look shabby in the Grand Bristol; tidy but shabby. I can't decide whether it is cruel to wear silk, like leather and fur, and I'm feeling a bit ashamed. I've convinced myself that the silk worms are all kept in battery farms and force-fed with mulberry leaves to produce miles and miles of silk. I'm sure silk worms just want to have fun.

Soldier has been getting much bolder of late and often comes for a stroke or a rub, but it has to be on his terms. In fact he is quite prepared to push Tiger out of the way. This causes great resentment because Tiger is so jealous and is not prepared to share my attentions and she sulks. Sometimes I have to sit on the ground, between them stroking a different cat with each hand simultaneously. Tiger is, and always will be, my favourite. We are kindred spirits, each yearning for the affection that only the other can give.

Again I have dreamt about them. I was marching purposefully out of the house clad all in denim with a knife in my inside jacket pocket. I think I was just slipping out to murder someone, but they were waiting for me, hidden behind the front wall, and surprised me with their shouting. Tiger and Soldier were both there and there was a third cat with them, a sort of phantom cat, that I couldn't actually see. I think it was probably Toffee, a pretty, brindled creature, who lives the other side of us. She is so shy you seldom see her. Tiger had even learnt to speak and I could hear her saying: "Hi," in a mewy sort of voice. She just has to outdo the others. I was so taken aback I forgot all about the murder. Someone was lucky.

I thought someone had dumped a Jag opposite the flats and I phoned the police. It's got two wheels on the kerb, the front tyre is nearly flat and the tax ran out months ago. It's been there ages. It's nearly ten years old and it's got a bit of damage, but it's still very beautiful in its metallic mid-green with its leather interior, alloy wheels and its 4.2 litre engine. My idea was that, if no one claimed it, I could have it. The policeman checked on his computer. The owner isn't local, but the car hasn't been stolen. He suggested I wait a couple of weeks and then write to see if I can buy it. I'd like that, purring along in a Jag and swooping past lesser cars, but I don't suppose I'll do anything about it. Who knows how much work it would need to have done and what would that would all cost? I can see it from the roof garden... it's still there.

Part Nine

It feels strange going away on holiday at the age of forty-one with my mother and sister, even though we have been three times before. As I said previously it's not what I would really choose, but probably they wouldn't either. We all have such different expectations of our holiday that they are not always easily accommodated when we are together. Can each of us find what we are hoping for in the Grand Bristol in Stresa? We must make the most of it.

We were up at five and had checked in at Gatwick by half past seven, but the flight was delayed an hour. It only takes an hour and a half to Milan and we were at the hotel by mid-afternoon. It was quite hot and very humid. The lake is beautiful, set in the lower reaches of the Alps. It looks quite clean, but sometimes you can smell it and I don't think I'll risk going in. Most people seem to use the hotel pools. The grass is green and lush and, although they are always watering it, it suggests to me that they have a fair amount of rain. There are flowers everywhere, in borders, beds, tubs, window boxes. Along the lakeside is a long wide promenade, also with shrubs and trees, where you can have a drink or an ice cream. The village of Stresa lies away from the road which runs beside the promenade. It's a maze of interlocking, narrow, cobbled streets with all sorts of interesting little shops. In the small main square are cafés with tables and umbrellas. Away from the main road it is quiet.

The hotel overlooks the lake and is about a quarter of an hour's walk from the centre of the village, which is a bit of a drag in the heat of the day. The lake is only four kilometres wide but there is often a haze and the dark grey clouds over the mountains when we arrived looked menacing. The hotel is very large and not too grand; it's comfortable, elegant and very modern. Everything is electronic and most of the facilities are controlled by a touch-sensitive control panel on the headboard of the bed: radio, window blind, lights, door, even the maid. There is no key; I have a card, like a credit card, which I place in a slot outside to open the door. This card also doubles up as a credit card for ordering drinks at the bar. There are two telephones in the room, one by the bed and, to save the four star guests from embarrassment, one by the toilet. Downstairs at reception they can tell on their computer if you have left your window open; do they also know when I'm on the toilet? In the cloakroom off the foyer the water starts to run automatically when you stand at the hand basin even if you are only combing your hair. We paid a large supplement for the single rooms, but they are very small and there isn't even a table in mine. I am sitting on my bed in my underpants writing this. I asked at reception if they would remove the bar and the television, which I don't want, and give me a little table instead, explaining that I liked to write. They weren't helpful at all, they made a great Italian fuss and I wished I hadn't asked. Still no table.

I was charged seven thousand lire (three pounds fifty) at the bar for a glass of wine before dinner when we arrived. This seemed exorbitant, but I didn't know what to expect so I have followed it up with the courier. I thought about the Hare and Hounds where we had paid less than that for our Sunday lunch. Today it was only three thousand. Soon they will be paying me. The evening meal is excellent and the young waiters charming, but four courses are really too much for me. I could make a meal of the antipasti alone.

I should be all right here; there are two big swimming pools, one indoor and one outdoor, both quite chilly, but at least one of my main needs is catered for and I feel comfortable in my room playing with the controls. There is plenty of room to sit around in the foyer and outside, but, knowing Eleanor, we'll be kept on the go. It's a shame that the people at reception weren't more friendly and helpful when we arrived, but I shall just ignore them. They would be much happier if there were no guests in the hotel to cause them aggravation, no requests for tables, but they have my sympathy. I've always thought schools would be pleasanter places without children.

All different nationalities are staying here; I've heard English, German and French as well as Italian. This evening we were commiserating with a Belgian lady who had been in tears over the death of King Baudouin.

Sunday

It always takes me a while to become accustomed to my new surroundings when I go away and I usually wish I hadn't come. This morning when I woke up I couldn't help thinking to myself that it was time for me to die. The knowledge of my infection makes each day seem like a struggle to survive. It would be easier to give up the fight, but I hope I never will.

In the morning we met the courier, Chris Ellis, a very pleasant young Englishman married to a local girl, who told us about the various trips and excursions and warned us about different pitfalls. There seems to be so much to do here; Eleanor and my mother will love it. After a pizza in the square we went to the botanical gardens in the grounds of the Villa Pallavicino, where there is also a little zoo. Some of the animals are quite tame and wander round freely. I stroked a llama, several goats and a deer. The llama seemed very affectionate and quite daft. One of the goats tried to chew Eleanor's floral print skirt until she batted it off with the brochure and he made a meal of that instead.

Before dinner we went to the pool for a swim and I saw a very attractive French guy. He was nut-brown, wearing white trunks, with his hair swept back from his forehead. Totally and devastatingly French, he just oozed sex from every pore. I realised then that a part of me has already died, probably killed off by my medication. All I am able to do is look and remember. I was close to tears as I sat drinking my wine before dinner. Why can't anyone do anything about this bloody virus? I am only forty-one, I'm not ready to die and I still want to have sex. My mind says yes, but my body says no.

Monday

I didn't sleep so well last night, but woke up feeling more cheerful and more hopeful. We visited Lake Orta, which is about ten miles west of Maggiore. The village lies at the tip of a peninsula which reaches out into the lake. Surrounded by wooded hills, the traffic-free centre was quiet and peaceful. We sat in a café at the water's edge with the water almost lapping round our feet, watching the housemartins skimming over the lake. It was just so beautiful. The lake is only one kilometre wide and, facing the village, just a few minutes' ride away by taxi boat, is the tiny island of San Giulio, only three hundred metres long by one hundred and sixty wide. The basilica contains a glass-sided silver shrine with the relics of San Giulio who came to the island from Aegina in the fourth century and converted the inhabitants to Christianity.

On the way back we stopped at the gigantic statue of San Carlo Borromeo, Cardinal Archbishop of Milan in the sixteenth century, which looks out over the lake. The name Borromeo first appeared when the pope named a member of the family 'Buono Romeo' and this was then contracted to Borromeo. Since the twelfth century the Borromeans have owned not only the three main islands in Lake Maggiore but also much of the land surrounding the lake and the castles beside it. One has the impression that the whole lake once belonged to them. They had it all wrapped up, politics, religion. It was an absolute power base.

Driving back along the lake to Stresa we passed the holiday villas of the Branca and Martini families. I shall never forget Orta.

We had a swim when we got back and I saw the French guy again. He's obviously interested. I feel I can't let him know I am too. With my infection it is too difficult and with my medication I probably couldn't respond which would be embarrassing. I shan't mention him again because it upsets me too much.

I've definitely got the barman rattled, I gave him five thousand lire for the wine and he gave me three thousand back by mistake.

Eleanor had a migraine and retired early. She thinks she may have become dehydrated. I ought to be drinking bottled water, but I can't be bothered and anyway I like the water here and it seems to agree with me.

Tuesday

A lightning tour of the three lakes, Maggiore, Lugano and Como. It is terribly important to remain completely passive on these long coach tours in order to enjoy them. We drove up the west side of Maggiore passing through the village of Cannero where, for fifteen years, pirates had inhabited the little island and terrorised the people. Apparently, the nudists have now taken over from them. We crossed the border into Switzerland and stopped at the top of the lake in Locarno for an hour. It's quite obvious that the Italians regard this area as belonging to them and it really is practically indistinguishable from Italy. It just happens to be in Switzerland. The international film festival was due to start in two days' time and preparations were being made. Prices were going up by the minute. I looked out for a woman running around in her knickers, but Madonna obviously hadn't arrived yet.

We drove on to Lugano for a three hour stop. It was busy, bustling and beautiful. We went into a very old church, la Chiesa degli Angeli, and saw a very fine early sixteenth century fresco of the Passion, painted by Bernardino Luini, a pupil of da Vinci. After lunch we sat in the shade in the park on the promenade with its magnificent flowers until it was time to get the coach.

Our next stop was Como, a big industrial city. The enormous cathedral, which had taken four centuries to complete, had some remarkable tapestries and paintings, some again by Luini, but it was so dark you could barely see them. You could put five hundred lire in a slot to have them illuminated, but we didn't have any change. Nor did anyone else, so it seemed. What I liked most were the small stained-glass windows round the altar which were so bright they looked like transparencies. Having seen the cathedral I was exhausted. The temperature in Como was over thirty degrees in the shade and still rising. We sat in a café by the lake until it was time to return. Back in Stresa it was spotting with rain.

Wednesday

I have found it quite impossible to sleep in this hotel so far. Apart from the first night when, exhausted by the journey, I fell immediately into a heavy sleep, I haven't slept well. First I tried with the shutter down and woke early feeling suffocated, then, last night, I left the shutter up and the windows wide open and woke at first light.. before even the dustmen arrived, the deliveries started and the coaches started up their engines spewing diesel fumes into my room. I shall make my last bid tonight; blind down, windows shut, air conditioning on. Nor is it possible to rest in the afternoon. My room is opposite the service lift which grinds continually up and down and where the maids clatter about with empty bottles from people's rooms and dump the bedding. Last night as I sat here on my bed with the windows wide-open I was visited by a hornet. It was quite frightening.

Today we went up the Mottarone (one thousand metres) by funicular railway. In the guide book this constitutes a day off. Stresa is two hundred and five metres above sea level. We stopped half way up to go to the Alpine garden. Most of the flowers had finished, but the view of the lake with the three islands and Baveno and Pallanza was superb. At the top we had quite a steep climb to get to the summit. I wasn't sure my legs would be up to it. I was puffing and blowing and kept having to stop. It was very hazy, but we could make out Maggiore and Orta. On a clear day you can see seven lakes, Monte Rosa and Milan. There were all kinds of pretty wayside flowers and butterflies. While we were having our meal the thunderclouds came and the waiter forecast rain in one hour, but by then we were safely back in Stresa. I didn't like the funicular; it made me feel queasy.

Thursday

We spent the morning in Stresa looking round the little shops and buying presents. This was shopping on a scale even I can enjoy. In the afternoon we went on a tour of the Borromean islands. These are not far from the shore and very close together. It only takes five minutes to reach them. First we visited Isola Madre, the mother island, where the Borromean children were sent to escape from the plague in Milan. The courier told us that the island had been artificially constructed where only a rock had been. We walked round the gardens with their exotic plants and trees and went into the villa where they had lived. There were enormous collections of dolls and puppets (some quite grotesque) and toys to keep them amused. The rain started to pour down as we were waiting for the boat to take us to Isola Bella, beautiful island. This was too beautiful for words to describe, both the palace and the gardens. Napoleon and Josephine had stayed here and in 1935 the Stresa agreement was signed here by MacDonald, Mussolini and Laval in an attempt to stop Germany rearming. Outside on the lawns were all-white albino peacocks and peahens strutting about, flirting with one another and showing off their offspring to the tourists. The centrepiece of the gardens is a large stone structure with statues, pillars and huge shells which is surmounted by a unicorn; behind this the terraced gardens fall away in ten tiers. Too beautiful even to imagine. Everywhere you could see the family motto 'humilitas', humility. It was even spelt out in flowers in the garden.

My legs hadn't recovered from the Mottarone and we seemed to be constantly climbing up and down. It was unbearably humid and I felt fit to drop. It was a relief then to get to the Isola Pescatori, fishermen's island, where we could find more shade among the old houses. There are about eighty people living there and they are all expected to marry another islander. When they die they are brought back to the island to be buried in the little churchyard behind the eleventh century church. It was here also in the Verbano Hotel that MacDonald, Mussolini and Laval had stayed.

Friday

I was talking to Luciano, the shifty barman, last night and asked him what happened to Stresa in the winter. Apparently all the hotels close down apart from the five star Grand Hotel et des Isles Borromées. The hotel staff make their way to the skiing villages for the winter season or some even come to London. He is lucky; his parents own a bar in Domodossola and he goes and helps them.

My mother and sister have gone to Milan today. I decided not to go because my legs are still very tired and I didn't fancy traipsing round Italy's second largest city in this heat. Also it is the ferragosto (August holiday) and most places, shops and factories are shut for the month while the Italians take their holidays.

I went back to Stresa this morning and walked the whole length of the promenade taking pictures. After a cappuccino in a bar on the front I went into the centre and continued my shopping. For myself I bought a nice pair of soft leather shoes for fifteen pounds. Some of the shop keepers recognised me from yesterday and called out: 'Buongiorno'. It was very busy and I discovered that it was market day. I had a lot of fun and got some quite good photographs. I had a little conversation with the waiter at the Ristorante Nazionale- where we had eaten before. He seemed to think it was good that I was having a day off from the women. I returned to the hotel laden like a pack-horse.

I have managed the Italian quite well, I did a year's study at university, but thought I had forgotten it all. In fact I remember things I didn't realise I knew. The Italians are all so pleasant, helpful and friendly, even those at reception now. They help out when my Italian fails me either with English or smiles and gestures.

I tried to rest again this afternoon, but it was just as noisy as before and I think I must ask for a quieter room.

I am sitting now in my new room writing this at a table. The only drawback is that the light is so poor. My mother and sister are back from Milan after a fairly exhausting day. Apparently there was no sign of ferragosto and business seemed to be being conducted normally. As I was caressing my new shoes admiringly this evening I found a label: Made in China.

Saturday/Sunday

The opera at Verona - Aida. What a spectacle, but never again. Verona is one hundred and fifty miles from Stresa and so the coach picked us up at three o'clock in the afternoon. There was a small delay as the people from the next hotel didn't turn up. We arrived at the amphitheatre just before seven and had to wait for the guide to collect our tickets. The gates opened at seven fifteen and we were advised to go in promptly although the opera didn't actually start until nine o'clock.

It was very hot, thirty-one degrees, and the amphitheatre was packed with over twenty thousand people. It was ghastly having to step round, between and over people to get to our places. All I could think about was the germs, but I was glad of my inflatable cushion, water bottle and wet flannel. I sat and read the synopsis and at nine o'clock it started.

It was magnificent in every way: the stage which comprised about a quarter of the whole amphitheatre, the sphinxes, the columns with their hieroglyphics, the costumes. It was outrageously extravagant, which is what opera is all about for me. The singing was superb, some voices better than others, of course. At the end of each scene there were great ovations as the set was changed.

Apart from the final scene with Radames and Aida entombed together and Amneris lying on their tomb full of remorse, the highlight for me was the triumphant return from battle after the capture of Amonasro. What magnificence. There were hundreds of people on stage: the Pharaoh and his cortège and Amneris, Amonasro and the captured Ethiopians and, of course, Radames, the hero, leader of the troops. There were horses, soldiers, trumpeters, troupes of dancers, ballet dancers, men with lighted torches and gold animals. A spectacle never to be surpassed.

The end finally came at a quarter past one. It really had been an ordeal in the great heat with all those people. There was a rush and a scramble to get out and I managed to strike a German woman a glancing blow to the side of the head with my camera. She wasn't very pleased. It was half an hour's walk to the coach and we set off for Stresa at just before two o'clock. We arrived back some time after five and rang for the night watchman. There was no response so we climbed over the fence into the hotel grounds and were about to make our way up the fire escape when he appeared. It had been an evening to be enjoyed retrospectively.

Monday

On our excursion to Verona we met a very nice couple from Jersey. Andrew and Carole had driven down from Fréjus in their convertible scarlet BMW M3 with its air conditioning, black leather seats and flared wheel arches, one of only two hundred ever made. It was Andrew who had suggested, as we were climbing over the fence at five o'clock in the morning, that it was our chance to beat the Germans to the sunbeds. As my sister and my mother were going to Venice for the day and I had cried off again because of the very early start, they had invited me to come out with them in the car. They hadn't been to Orta and I was longing to go back. All I knew about Jersey was what I had seen on the television in 'Bergerac': wealthy people involved in shady business deals, garden and dinner parties. I was thrilled to be going out with them and to have a ride in the BMW. The M3 is a seriously fast motor car.

After the violent storm over the lake the night before the air was fresh and it was clearer than it had been all holiday. The early morning light was beautiful and we had some spectacular views of both lakes as we drove over the hills and through wooded valleys. Sitting in the back of the BMW was exhilarating but also quite chilly so Carole and I swapped over half way there. Orta was as lovely as before, but this time we had all day to amble round looking in the little shops, and to visit the island again. We had our lunch on the terrace of a restaurant built out over the lake, and covered in vines hanging with bunches of ripening grapes. It was delightful. Andrew and Carole, who told me that they had got engaged within two hours of meeting, have a son called Matthew. We had dinner together in the evening. I enjoyed their conversation, their company and the car. They were warm, generous people with a sense of fun and, after twenty years together, clearly still very much in love. After dinner Andrew introduced me to Amaretto, a marvellous almond liqueur.

Tuesday

Our intention had been to visit the botanical gardens at the Villa Tarranto, but we got off the boat at Pallanza for a cup of coffee and decided it looked a nice little place to explore. Eleanor, in any case, prefers shops to plants and my legs are tired of walking anywhere. I am all right on the level, but uphill still exhausts me. We walked along the promenade lined with oleanders and magnolia trees with enormous blooms and saw the San Giovanni island, which is reserved for the exclusive use of the Borromean family; it is also known as the Toscanini island since the time when he lived there. We could hear the students practising in the music school.

Before lunch, while Eleanor and my mother were still looking round the shops, I sat down on a bench in the shade, where an Italian lady was reading her newspaper. After a while she turned to me and complained that she felt chilly. She'd lived in Pallanza for ten years and said the climate suited her. She told me I must go to Rome and complimented me on my Italian. She had done all the talking. Apart from one short sentence I had just agreed with what she was saying.

With all the trips we've been on I feel we have perhaps rather neglected the lake itself. This is a shame; I enjoyed our trip to Pallanza. It was a pretty place, but I felt glad we were staying in Stresa; it's bigger and there's more to do.

It was that evening also that I met Alberto. He was about two years old and had been entrusted to his sister to be taken downstairs. He saw me in the lift, turned on his heel and fled down the corridor. He was a mass of fair curls and was wearing long white shorts down to his ankles. He couldn't quite keep up with his legs which gave the impression that the shorts had a momentum of their own and were propelling him on at headlong speed.

Wednesday

It is a quarter past eleven and I have packed my case and shut it. The others have gone on one final trip and I walked into Stresa with Carole and Andrew, who are also leaving today. I bought one or two last presents and then went and sat at the end of the harbour wall next to the statue of the Madonna. She had her back to me, but I touched the hem of her robe and asked her to help me. I shall have lunch. The lunch here is even better than the evening meal. I have my eye on the macaroni followed by the veal escalope with ham and cheese. Then, after a snooze in the shade, I shall have time for one last swim. I shall wave goodbye to Fabiana, an eleven year old girl who lies on the edge of the pool watching me swim up and down before jumping in and splashing around with her friend while I watch them. Then the coach comes to pick us up at five o'clock ready for our flight at eight.

I don't want to go home; it is very beautiful here and seems to become more so every day. I shall miss the hotel and the young woman at reception who seems now to have taken a shine to me. She even confided to me that she also writes, when she feels sad. When I am back I shall have to face up to my situation again. What am I going back to? Nothing, I can spend another month finishing my writing, but what then? I have no job, no lover, no future.

We arrived back at about half past ten and Tiger came out to meet us; she always appears when she hears my car. She was desperate for affection and I was happy to supply it. I enjoyed the holiday; I think we all did, it certainly did me some good by taking me away from Stanmore and the clinic. In addition, we had really got on quite well together.

It was my first time in Italy and if I have another holiday it is where I shall return to. The Italians struck me as intelligent and sophisticated. They have a multi-billion pound tourist industry and they treat their visitors with grace, charm and style. In other countries I've visited the people seemed to be resentful of the tourists and to consider catering for them demeaning, losing sight of the revenue they were bringing in. The climate was hot without being harsh and the hotels, restaurants and coaches are all air conditioned so you can always escape from the heat. England seems so gloomy, so dreary by comparison. The emphasis there is far more on enjoyment.

While we were away I noticed that my mother seemed to find it difficult to talk to me and addressed herself always to my sister and confided in her.

When we went out I knew they were both monitoring me. Have I got my bag? Where's my camera? Eleanor, I felt, was always looking over my shoulder, ready to correct me should I make the least mistake. It is probably their way of showing their love and concern for me, but their anxiety makes me want to explode. When I feel I'm being watched so closely I am apt to be clumsy and make mistakes. Then I start to feel stupid and get cross. I want to tell them that they would do better to attend to themselves, that I am not their responsibility, that I am not a little boy anymore. I need to be loved, not monitored.

My mother attaches herself to my sister and seems to be happy to go along with whatever pleases Eleanor. Eleanor is more complicated. We got on quite well together like we used to before our father died, but she so often seems cross, either with herself or with my mother or me and she finds it impossible to conceal her irritation and frustration. She has to be off somewhere every day, otherwise she regards it as failure, not to have exploited the holiday to the full. She is not content just to enjoy being there. She had two migraines while we were away. Sometimes she is terribly tense and you just need to look at her to know she's going to get it. On the second occasion I told her in the morning that she needed to slow down and calm down. She pushes herself too hard and then, instead of thinking that she ought to take it easy, to relax a little, she just gets cross with herself. She must learn to be kinder to herself and then she will be more tolerant of other people's shortcomings.

What is most important for me, however, is that they are happy doing everything together and knowing that they will be all right when I'm no longer around.

And what about me? I really did enjoy myself and I blame it partly on the virus that I didn't enjoy the other holidays more. This time I was not so exhausted going away and felt more relaxed. I had more energy and felt fitter, sharper, more confident. In fact, I felt at least ten years younger than on the previous holidays; it was always such a struggle for me before, I think I have to attribute this improvement in part to the AZT.

I missed Julian while I was away. I had no one to share my thoughts with. My mother and sister are not really on my wavelength and are either not listening to or interested in what I might have to say. However, I didn't feel excluded by their alliance to the extent I had previously. They treated me with more consideration and their expectations of me seemed to have changed. They didn't look to me to substitute for my father to the extent that I felt they had done before, and they made fewer demands on me which I felt unable to fulfil.

I need to have some space while we are away and the days when they went to Milan and Venice and on a boat trip across the lake allowed me to catch up with my writing and to take stock. Also I was able to have some adventures and some fun on my own.

I thought I was getting a throat infection a couple of times, once after our ascent of the Mottarone and one very hot afternoon, but it never came to anything very much. Presumably the powerful antibiotics I'm taking for the Xenopi helped me to fight it off. Otherwise I had no problems apart from my legs. I think I was probably using muscles I don't normally use. All the walking I do is on the flat; there are no mountains in Stanmore.

I noticed that eating was a bit of a problem. I feel hungry, but I am quickly sated and then I start to struggle and am terribly slow. Most people have finished and I'm not even half way through my meal. Somehow my heart's not really in it. I think sometimes that the food would be better deployed feeding the starving in the developing world than keeping me alive.

I hope it isn't my last holiday and that we can all go away again together next year.

Part Ten

I was back in the clinic for my next appointment within twenty-four hours of the plane touching down. Dr Kapembwa looked at the colour of my skin and said I was catching him up. Then he announced that he felt the time was right to consider combination therapy again, now that I had been on AZT for more than six months. He wanted me back in three weeks' time to discuss it with him. This was a complete surprise as I thought he intended keeping me just on the AZT. I was pleased; it seemed to indicate that he had taken note of my letter and that he was prepared to be bold in my treatment.

I don't have strong views any more on the benefits of combination therapy and don't hold out any false hopes, it has already been tried without notable success. Progress in medical science is always painstakingly slow and I realise that even this won't defeat the virus though it may, or may not, keep me going a bit longer. I am prepared to go along with it if Dr Kapembwa wants me to give it a go. If he can learn something from it, that is sufficient justification for me.

My holiday may have done me a power of good while I was away, but again I felt lonely and depressed when I was back. It had been a treat not to have to cook and clean and shop, to have my bed made and my room cleaned. It had been interesting and stimulating to visit all the new places, to meet new people and to say a few words in Italian. Most important perhaps was that I had had almost constant company.

After my visit to the clinic I felt immediately thrust back into the rather dreary routine which was dominated by my infection with nothing very much to take my mind off myself. As I had feared, I felt my life had no purpose other than to continue the battle against the virus and to try to keep well; this seemed totally unproductive. I had my writing, but that was nearing completion and, in any case, my depression was making me disillusioned with the whole undertaking, making me wish I'd never started.

I saw Eva once before she went on holiday to the South of France. We spent a very nice afternoon together in her garden. There seemed to be so much to say on both sides. I told her how I felt that I had no future any more, but she reminded me that I still had myself and that was the most important thing. She showed me a letter she had received inviting her to an international congress in Zurich in 1995 and we talked about the possibility of her presenting a paper on me and my infection. I told her I would be more than willing to cooperate and so she decided to send off a submission. She is going to call it 'Hanging on and letting go'. If it is accepted I shall be tempted to go too. She can use me as a visual aid, a patient with AIDS, and then I'll sit at the back flogging my book. She had picked me another little bunch of flowers which she gave me along with my birthday present. I wished she hadn't been going away or, at least, that I could have gone with her and taken my writing with me. Peter was also away in France.

Still, it was my other friends who came to the rescue. I saw Julian again and we resumed the old-established Friday evening routine. Lesley, who had moved from her flat a couple of months previously into a maisonette about a mile away, came round and we had a good chat. Then I went round to Mike and Mike for a meal. My spirits lifted a little.

The reports on the Berlin conference made fairly dismal reading. Still no headway seems to have been made against the virus itself even though other treatments are becoming ever more sophisticated. One really could believe that AIDS is a cull, a scourge sent by an angry if not a wicked god. We are all helpless in the face of it.

There was the outcome of the Concorde study and the discouraging results in the first trial of AZT and ddC. The TAT inhibitor had proved to be ineffective and had been abandoned and convergent combination therapy hadn't worked, the virus having failed to mutate in the way predicted in laboratory studies. There was general disappointment at the limited usefulness of the drugs currently available, and activists were recommending that the best hope was to divert funding from further trials into basic scientific research which might lead to the discovery of more effective treatments.

There were other, newer drugs, like the protease inhibitor, which seek to attack the virus in different ways and there was talk of antisense technology, but the problem remained of getting adequate levels of the drug absorbed into the body and preventing it from being broken down in the bloodstream.

While we were away a rather strange report hit the headlines of *The Sunday Times* which Eva had cut out and sent to me. Some scientists were claiming that the HIV tests, which detect antibodies to the virus in the blood, are scientifically invalid, that neither of the two main tests had been adequately checked for accuracy and that they were incapable of determining whether people are really infected with HIV. A positive result may be triggered in people with other conditions such as malaria, malnutrition, TB, multiple sclerosis and warts. Even the flu jab can produce the same effect. The longer the immune system has been weakened, by whatever cause, the more likely people are to give a positive result.

In the same report it stated that there is a growing number of scientists making their voices heard who believe that HIV is not the true cause of AIDS. They say that there is no proof that people labelled HIV positive are infected with such a retrovirus. They maintain that it is a false correlation which has been found between HIV antibodies and AIDS, that there is no mechanism by which HIV could do the damage attributed to it. There is no animal test, no cure, no vaccine, no virus activity to support the view that HIV causes AIDS. There is nothing in terms of conventional virus disease argument to support the theory. The whole hypothesis rests on the correlation with antibodies and now even that seems to be in doubt in view of the unreliability of the HIV tests.

It is a strange but interesting idea and cannot be disregarded. At the least I find it confusing. So, if not an HIV retrovirus, what is causing the damage to people's immune systems? I find it difficult to believe that the experts have all been barking up the wrong tree, but it would explain why no real headway has been made in discovering any effective medication.

It was food for thought and, however far-fetched, it did make me wonder. Here was I, who had always been susceptible to warts and verrucas, who had a mycobacterial infection akin to TB, who had had a 'flu jab and had tested positive. I wasn't suggesting that I didn't have the virus, though it did cross my mind to retest; it just seemed that there must be some connection between all these things other than the virus, whether or not it existed. I supposed it must be the weakened immune system.

At the end of August a new trial is to start in London, using forty male volunteers, of thalidomide, which is now used to treat leprosy. It is believed to block a protein which HIV uses to infect new cells. Researchers believe that it may be able to alleviate the symptoms of AIDS and slow or even halt its progress. This sounded to me like clutching at straws.

I felt I was lucky to be having another birthday at all and didn't want a great fuss to be made like it might be my last, but I was disappointed that Julian hadn't suggested that we should go out for a meal. I always cook him a birthday meal; I'd even managed this year. Apart from Friday evenings when he comes round he is never willing for us to go out together anymore. I think the routine he prides himself on is threatening to take over his life. He is always 'doing other things', his chores or buying clothes. He is trapped living at home with his parents, and keeping up appearances. He is not able to live his own life or even allow me to ring him up at home. David is much the same; he rings me quite often now, but is not prepared for us to meet up. I had so hoped to see him one more time this side of the grave. I'm not sure what frightens him most: me or the infection. Peter is far more enterprising; he has loads of interests.

I spent the weekend with my mother who, after the holiday, was feeling equally flat. In fact, as if to emphasise this, she had tripped on a manhole cover in Leatherhead and fallen flat on her face. I hadn't realised how badly she had hurt herself. She looked a dreadful mess and had been very shaken by the fall. She had bruising all round one eye and down her cheek, and her forehead, nose and chin were all scratched. She had been too embarrassed to go out and when I arrived home there was no little present for me and the cupboard was almost bare, but she had made a lovely apple tart.

On the Saturday, my birthday, I persuaded her to come down to Paddy's, for lunch. He is such a gentleman I think she forgot all about her embarrassment. In the afternoon we sat on the beach in the warm sunshine and I had a swim in my underpants. I had brought a towel just in case, but my trunks were in Stanmore. The sea was warm, much warmer than the hotel pool in Stresa and I have always loved to swim in the sea though I know that it is not wise for me to do so anymore.

I understood that weekend better than before my mother's fear of growing old. She has always been a vigorous, independent woman and could not bear to become incapacitated. I so wish I could assure her that I will be there for her and that she needn't be afraid. And how will Eleanor fare when we are both gone?

The following week I went round to see a friend from school. She is the only one of my colleagues who has kept in regular telephone contact with me. The others seem to have forgotten about me except perhaps for Peter, Head of Sixth Form, who has come round to see me a couple of times. She and her husband have two adopted children, brothers, whom I have seen from time to time over the last thirteen years and watched grow up. They are now eighteen and nineteen. In the last five years they have had dreadful problems with both boys, but most of all with their younger son. He has been in all sorts of trouble. He has on occasions threatened his parents and not infrequently inflicted harm on himself. No one seems to know what the matter is with him, but he is very disturbed and just seems to lose control. I have never witnessed the negative side. He has always impressed me with his good manners and charm. He is a good looking boy and always sharply dressed. He is bright, affectionate and good with children. He has been on all manner of treatment and is now locked away in a mental hospital under a section order.

When I arrived his mother told me that he had been ringing her to see if I was there yet, so I suggested to her that we go and visit him. He was thrilled to see us. He gave his mum a long, heartfelt hug and I could see immediately how very much he loves her despite the awful trouble he has caused. There are three types of ward at the hospital, open, secure and closed. They had been keeping him in the secure ward until he had broken a window with his hand, when they had moved him to the closed ward where he was being held together with other patients, some of whom had a criminal record. He had also somehow forfeited his parole and wasn't allowed to go swimming. He was on fairly heavy medication and couldn't always find his words; he had obviously been crying and his hand was bandaged as a result of the glass.

He was very grateful for the cigarettes I'd brought him. Fortunately I had also taken some photographs of my holiday with me to show my friend. I don't know how we would have spent the time otherwise or what we would have talked about. You could see his imagination working as he looked at each one closely and intently, and he and his mother sat and reminisced about the holiday they had spent in Italy many years ago with their Italian friends. The half hour we had intended staying with him turned unnoticed into an hour, but then he had to go and have his tea. It was a painful and emotional farewell when we left. Outside I realised that for the first time in nine months I had been able to put myself and my infection out of my mind completely.

I missed my next appointment at the clinic, though I did, of course, ring up to cancel it. I was cruising up the River Arun to Amberley Castle in something akin to a motorised bath-tub when I should have been seeing Dr Kapembwa to discuss the combination therapy. It was the first week of September and the forecast had been good so I had gone down to Felpham to enjoy the last of the Summer.

Paddy was on form. When is he not? But business had been slow and he was a bit depressed. We had several trips out together and he cheered up. I was very touched that most of his friends made the effort to see me, coming for lunch or going out for a drink. I'm sure it is frightening meeting someone with AIDS when you don't know how ill they are or what to expect. Judging from the conversation they all have, or have had, a far higher risk lifestyle than ever I did.

The sea was much colder now, too cold for comfort, and so, after the first day when I braved the freezing cold water, the sharp stones, the chill East wind, the seaweed and the flies and emerged after only a few minutes shuddering with cold I decided to swim in the hotel pool. My appetite seemed much better down there and I could happily pack away three cooked meals a day. Perhaps it was the sea air or perhaps the problem lies with my cooking when I'm at home, which is boring and unimaginative.

I met a German lady who mistook me for a priest. I was wearing some black trousers and the grey sweatshirt which exposed about an inch of my white T-shirt, making it look like a cleric's collar. She started to confide in me. I told her I wasn't a priest, but it made no difference. She obviously needed one and had decided that I would do. I just listened to her troubles; she was very grateful.

There is a row of what can only be described as shacks along the front at Felpham. These tiny properties appear to form the first line of defence against the sea. They seem no more substantial than beach-huts. One wave or one gust of wind and you'd think they'd be gone, flying through the air over the South Downs, but they've been there for years. Wooden or prefabricated and resting on piles, some are pristine, others dilapidated. These are in fact freehold properties and one was for sale. 'Seaside' boasted two double bedrooms, a lounge, dining room, kitchen and bathroom. Where all these rooms were I had no idea, it looked so small from the outside. It wasn't cheap, but if I had the money I'd get it and spend most of my time down there by the sea. There is always something to do at the seaside regardless of the weather. You can sit in the sun on the prom or fight your way through the wind and rain to the Boathouse for a cup of coffee. On a clear night you can watch the moon reflected in the sea.

Certainly the people are friendlier than in Stanmore and generally smile and acknowledge you as you walk along. There is nothing to do here and so many of the people seem mistrustful and unfriendly. I toyed with the idea of selling my flat and moving down there. I can, after all, die of AIDS anywhere; there are no restrictions, I think though that I do not want to transfer my treatment to another hospital and leave Dr Kapembwa and his team who have looked after me so well. Nor is the property probably robust enough to live in comfortably in the winter.

If I come out of this alive I think I would like to live in a little house on the coast and have my own little boat with an outboard motor.

I was starting to feel bitter about what might have been, what I could have made of my life, if circumstances had been different, and I had been dwelling on old hurts, past disappointments and failures. I knew it was pointless and unproductive; I just couldn't help it. What mattered now was what I could make of the rest of my life. I resolved that I must try to regard this time as my retirement, albeit somewhat premature, and try to enjoy the time I had left.

I am still frightened of letting go of my job completely and it will be good when the link with school is finally severed and it is no longer an option to return, but I do feel guilty about drawing my pension and the invalidity benefit, feeling as good as I do. It is contrary to my expectation of what I should be doing at the age of forty-two.

Now that my health seems reasonably stable I feel that I should have an occupation and I decided that I might benefit from some professional advice. It had been a very great blow to me that it wasn't worth my while to go back to work. I hadn't even been certain that it was what I wanted, but it had seemed the ideal solution. It was what I am trained to do and, even though only part-time, it would have given me a purpose and represented a return to normality which I felt was important. I didn't feel ready to give up entirely and I felt I ought to be working.

Although I had been in touch with the Terrence Higgins Trust and Body Positive on the phone I hadn't actually been along to either. The nearest drop-in centre to me is Earl's Court and, although I had felt quite interested to go, it takes so long on the tube that it hadn't seemed worth the effort. I felt that now was perhaps the time to go along to the THT and talk to a trained counsellor. I also thought it might be profitable to meet other people with AIDS and find out what they are doing and how they are coping. I rang to make an appointment.

I spoke to one of the counsellors. He explained that they have a bank of some twenty-five people, trained professionals, who give up one day a week to work at the Trust. He took my number and told me that I would hear from someone within the next forty-eight hours. I had told him I wanted a man, someone older than me, if possible.

Twenty minutes later he rang back; he had decided to take me on himself. I am pinning a lot of hope on this interview. I am not looking for a replacement for Eva. I'm hoping to discover what the way ahead may be for me and sort myself out on a more practical level with someone who has experience of other people with HIV and knows the sorts of things they are doing.

My visit to the Terrence Higgins Trust was a total disaster, it took me a long time to get to Grays Inn Road, three different tubes but I did arrive just before eleven o'clock; there were tears in my eyes as I walked the last hundred yards.

I made myself a beaker of coffee and the counsellor came to fetch me from reception. Clutching his personal organiser, he was the very antithesis of the mature, ageing professional I was hoping to see; the wise old man, to whom I would have poured out my soul.

Could I smoke? What harm could it have possibly done to let me have a fag? I felt he was asserting himself unnecessarily. After the long tube journey I was dying for one. I was told it was a fire risk. I replied that after twenty years' practice I could usually get the ash in the ashtrays. I started to feel bolshie and knew that the session was doomed.

When we had spoken on the phone I had told him that I wanted some practical advice as to what I could do to make the most of the rest of my life. Particularly, I had told him that I wanted to know whether I could do any paid work without forfeiting my benefit. He knew also that I had been in analysis for twenty years.

He didn't know the answers to my questions any better than the newly-privatised DSS. He was just intent on counselling me, but I didn't want or need that, and really not with him. I just wanted a chat and a few pointers.

Here was another man who was intense and unsmiling and who stared at me (I think there is something definitely freakish in me). I looked around the room and examined the door frame a hundred times to avoid his staring eyes and occasionally gave him a rather forced, feeble smile. There were long silences during which he continued to try to penetrate me with his eyes. I felt sure that he wanted me to break down and cry.

He asked me all the pertinent questions and I trotted out all the well-worn answers, things I had already dealt with and have written about here. How did I feel about the infection? What did I think about crying? What support was I getting from the community (by which he meant the 'gay' community)? Could I join a group? He was concerned about my isolation in Stanmore. Could I move? Did I want a 'buddy'?

Some of these questions I found bizarre, but I took them seriously and answered as best I could, I should rather not have the infection. I sometimes cry when I feel sad. I didn't want to join a group. I'd been to one in the past and it wasn't for me. There were always bossy people in groups who thought that they knew best and tried to organise you and there were those who tried to monopolise proceedings. It was too much like school. I certainly didn't want to move and leave behind the few friends that I do have. And no, I didn't want a 'buddy'. I had my own friends without having to be allocated someone with whom I would probably have nothing in common.

After twenty minutes he was sitting on the very edge of his seat in his attempt to get through to me. I suppose I wasn't unresponsive, but I seemed to irritate him because I didn't respond in the way I was intended to. At the end he implied that I was not listening to him. I apologised and assured him I was, explaining that it was just my way and that actually I never missed anything. I was just feeling rather flat and sad. I didn't want to have this infection and I didn't want to be there. I would have felt more comfortable in a funeral parlour. We didn't get anywhere. It was a complete waste of time and did more harm than good.

Before I left I made an appointment to see someone in the Welfare Department who could guide me through the different benefits which are available, but I don't want benefits. I want to go out to work and earn my keep.

I was in tears as I arrived home, tears of exhaustion, frustration and disappointment. I felt that it was all my fault that it had been so unproductive. He wasn't a bad chap, but he had been the wrong person for me and hadn't handled me very skilfully. He lacked warmth and I could not respond to him. I need human beings, not experts, carers, counsellors, psychoanalysts or whatever. Too often they are trapped within their roles and it is not possible to relate to them as people. They have a rigid, inflexible approach and identify people by their problems, me by my infection. Eva is different. She is gentle and kind. We sit and talk like old friends and I pour out my sadness to her. She is wiser and she helps me to understand things I'm struggling with. Sometimes we disagree, sometimes we clash, but it doesn't matter; I know she is on my side. All I want are people who are kind and feeling, like the two coloured girls in reception who were answering the telephones. They both had warm smiles; I could have talked to them.

After a cup of tea and a rest I did my ironing so that the whole day wouldn't have been wasted. I must find my own answers, but I guess I knew that all along.

A couple of days later I woke up feeling a bit rough and stiff after the last of my hepatitis B injections and realised that the answer had been there all along and I hadn't seen it, perhaps because I hadn't been ready to see it. It was a way of giving something back to the hospital which had saved my life and cared for me, a way of repaying my debt of gratitude.

Without a job my life seemed to have fallen apart. I needed an occupation, something which I considered worthwhile, something which would take me out of the flat a couple of times a week and where I would meet people. Friends had suggested voluntary work; I could offer my services to the Terrence Higgins Trust or the Lighthouse and maybe even do some counselling. This didn't appeal at all. I didn't want AIDS to take over my life. There were other important things to do. I would have preferred to do a couple of hours in the Oxfam shop except that it was being run perfectly well by a gaggle of ageing Stanmore ladies who, I felt sure, wouldn't welcome a young interloper.

I rang Janet Chater. She has been marvellous, coming round and phoning up. She is full of good advice and I think she really cares about me. She had suggested that I might like to have a chat with Tony Andrews, the hospital chaplain, and I was to let her know if I wanted her to make an appointment for me. He seemed the right man to discuss my ideas with.

I intended to find out whether there was any educational provision for the long-stay patients in the children's ward. I could perhaps go in for a couple of hours and do something with them which was enjoyable and stimulating. At the very least I could read them a story. Then there were the old people, the undervalued in our society, the people with a wealth of knowledge and experience of life. They have discovered some of the answers that the rest of us are still struggling to find. Why we don't pay more attention to them is beyond my comprehension. There might be some who were alone in the world. I would enjoy visiting them if they would welcome it. And there were the dying. I could go in and hold their hands, both figuratively and literally.

There were other possibilities too. Stanmore Orthopaedic is only a couple of miles up the road. I knew that they employed teachers there. Elm Park Tertiary College is just over the road from me. Perhaps I could give a couple of German conversation classes; and there was, if all else failed, always that old school where they would welcome some extra support. There were plenty of things I could do which were worthwhile and rewarding. It would mean that I wouldn't be sitting at home dwelling on my health and waiting for something to go wrong.

Understandably I wasn't keen to return to the Terrence Higgins Trust after my last experience. I phoned my mum and suggested that we should meet for lunch. In that way my appointment wasn't the sole purpose of the day.

I put on a new jacket I had bought eighteen months previously and never worn, and a shirt and tie and left my flat midmorning. I had a cup of coffee in town and had a look round Burton's before making my way to the Kingsley Hotel. We had a good meal in pleasant surroundings. I was pleased to find that my mother was getting involved in a few things again. There were a couple of classes she was going to attend and she had gone back to the local Junior School to listen to the children reading. She always was an excellent teacher.

I left to get the tube at two o'clock; I was in a completely different frame of mind from my last visit. I felt good because I knew I looked good and I had enjoyed my lunch. The same two girls were in reception and they made me welcome. The counsellor I had seen on the previous occasion came in and recognised me and I shook his hand. I could see now why he had been the wrong person for me.

This time I went to see Colin Nee, the Welfare Manager. He was a businesslike young man and very knowledgeable about the different benefits which are available. He listened sympathetically to what I had to say and seemed to understand my dilemmas and uncertainties. As I have an AIDS diagnosis I am entitled to Disability Living Allowance. This benefit is unrelated to income or savings and would give me an extra seventy-five pounds a week. He fetched the form and we filled it in on the spot. I felt angry that no one had drawn my attention to this benefit. I had missed out on ten months; this was money I could have put to good use, but which couldn't now be backdated. This money is not charity. I have paid my National Insurance contributions for twenty years and it is my entitlement. Surely the Social Services had known that anyone with an AIDS diagnosis was entitled to this benefit and they should have checked that I was receiving it instead of telling me about services which I didn't yet require and hoped I never would. They had been all talk.

He didn't believe me when I told him that I would be fifteen hundred pounds a year worse off if I went back to work part-time, but he fetched his calculator and confirmed my calculation. We talked a little about whether I should go back. Obviously the money was not a consideration. Did I want to? Not particularly, I wasn't sure. He advised me not to go back unless I wanted to and felt confident that I would be able to manage. He felt that, if I returned and found it too much and had to give up, it would set me back.

I told him about my plan to do some voluntary work. He advised me not to take on too much, just a couple of sessions a week and stick with it for a month or more. I could increase the load then if I wanted to. He suggested that I could work for an AIDS charity, but I said that though I could probably do it and might well find it rewarding, I didn't want my life to be dominated by AIDS. He understood.

He was an extremely understanding young man and happy to sit and chat to me. He knew the answers to my questions and was full of sound, practical advice. He was obviously the man I should have seen from the start. I came away feeling positive and with a completely different perception of the Trust. It had certainly helped me today. It's just that I never wanted counselling; I find it intrusive.

After my interview I went along to Dillons and bought a couple of books I'd been after. I felt whacked as I sat in the tube on my way home, but I was going to Harrow Arts Centre that evening with Mike and Mike to see a play, it was a one-person play by Peter Flannery, acted by Guy Masterson, about an ex-professional goalkeeper. It was excellent, dynamic, moving, comic. He filled the theatre with his performance. I couldn't believe that he wasn't telling his own true story, it was so convincing.

It had been a super day, nice lunch, profitable interview, marvellous play. I couldn't help feeling that it all had something to do with my new jacket.

Eventually I saw Dr Kapembwa again to discuss the possible benefits of adding ddI as a second anti-viral drug to my treatment. I was still fairly certain in my mind that I must have been infected around 1979. If so, my own immune system hadn't done a bad job of staving off the infections until last year and I hoped secretly that I was perhaps infected with a less virulent strain of the virus. What I felt I needed was something which would help my immune system rather than take over from it, something to tip the balance of power away from the virus and back towards my immune system. I wondered whether it was wise to interfere with the combination of drugs I was on, which seemed to be working so well. In addition, there seemed to be no definitive evidence that ddI worked at all.

Dr Kapembwa also felt that there was nothing to be gained at this stage by adding another drug while my clinical status continued to improve, albeit more slowly now, and I was feeling so well. I think we were both happy to hold the ddI in reserve in case the AZT started to fail and to be guided by the old maxim 'leave well alone'.

We talked a little about Africa where, in certain parts, the infection is endemic. The Ugandan Asians don't get AZT. All they are given is a Bible.

I may have made it sound like I feel perfectly all right. This is misleading. I am in pretty good shape and my weight has stabilised at eleven and a half stone, but my CD4 count has fallen to thirty and I long sometimes to have my old body back, the willing, the uncomplaining. There is nothing seriously wrong at the moment. My lungs are now clear apart from the shadow which stubbornly persists, but there are niggling little things which are probably due to the medication I'm still taking for the Xenopi rather than to the virus. These problems are very minor and I have mentioned them all already in passing.

My bowels are still affected by the antibiotics and a few minutes after getting up in the morning I have to rush to the toilet and then again half an hour later and sometimes again. Fortunately this is not diarrhoea and after this I am fine for the day. I have occasional recurrences of thrush which I also believe are caused by the drugs. I itch, but I am most conscious of this at night and it occasionally prevents me from falling asleep. For the first five months after treatment began I woke very early, never later than about six o'clock. I would be wide awake and found it impossible to lie in bed. Having then got up so early I felt tired by midmorning and by lunch-time I was ready to go back to bed. I am sleeping later now and feeling better for it, but I still feel weary and have to rest most days.

My legs are not as strong as they used to be despite the exercise I've taken, walking and swimming. It is sometimes an effort climbing up all the stairs to the flat, but on other occasions, I can charge up two at a time. When I first went into hospital my feet felt slightly numb, like they didn't quite belong to me. I didn't mention it to the doctors at the time, I'm not sure why, I think I was just too frightened to. I imagined that they might have to amputate my feet. My overall improved fitness and the B_6 vitamin supplement I'm taking seem largely to have cured this problem and my feet feel like they belong properly to me again.

I feel most comfortable in my own familiar environment with my own routine where I can take my time and, if I need to, I can shut my eyes for half an hour. Away from the flat I still occasionally feel dopey and distracted and I'm not quite sure what I'm doing or what's going on.

I should rather that the Xenopi finished me off than the pneumonia. I don't like the pneumonia with the awful night sweats and high temperature. When I was in hospital I sometimes used to have to call the nurse during the night to change my bedding, which was drenched. In contrast, the Xenopi is a gentler, kinder illness which just makes me feel incredibly tired and weary. I hope that with one enormous yawn I will just fall asleep one day and never wake up.

Perhaps the worst things are the dreadful uncertainty, the not knowing what will happen or when it will happen, and the fear. Will I still be around at Christmas? Will I have another holiday? I don't know, I can't count on it. I imagine that the end will come relatively suddenly, as it did for Howard, that there will be no long period of decline. I am constantly on my guard against the infection, and it is never completely out of my mind for fear that it will creep up on me when my guard is down, just when I've started to forget about it.

I don't want to lose my sight or my mental powers. I don't want to watch the cancerous lesions spreading over my body. . I am frightened of all these things and more. What will happen to me when I can no longer fend for myself? Will I be able to have a little room in the Lister Unit where I can retain some measure of independence and dignity?

The time may come when Dr Kapembwa has done his best and I've played my part, but it has become too much to bear and life is no longer worth living, when it is time to die. I don't know when that may be, but I will know when the time comes. I think sometimes that I was meant to have died last December and so to have avoided all the fear and anguish which I am experiencing now. I don't really believe this and certainly I'm glad I survived. I think I was meant to see Orta.

In Dr Kapembwa's office I noticed a list of all the HIV patients showing whether they were symptomatic or not. I wonder how he feels knowing that all these people are going to die unless a cure is found.

As has perhaps been apparent, my infection has placed a very great strain on my relationships with people, particularly those I'm closest to. It has, of course, hit my immediate family hardest; my sister, who never lets you know what she is thinking or feeling, unless you have incurred her displeasure, and my mum who is rather depressive and who has found this all so hard to bear.

Their phone calls have resumed since we returned from Stresa, but they are not quite so frequent now. I am grateful for this for the daily calls left me feeling that my life wasn't my own any more and I became taciturn and uncommunicative. I felt that these phone calls had more to do with their needs than mine. They are both a bit lonely sometimes, as indeed am I, and they are looking for reassurance that they are not alone. Now I look forward to hearing from them. I don't have much to say. I don't do anything exciting or, if I do, I don't always want to share it with them. Sometimes it would, in any case, be inappropriate. It would be so much better if Eleanor didn't live so far away and we could all meet up more easily. The telephone isn't really an adequate substitute.

People have not been able to keep the knowledge of my infection to themselves. This is understandable; it was a great shock for them too, but sometimes I wonder just how many people do know now and who they are. It doesn't really bother me, I have been lucky. I haven't been shunned by anyone and have detected very little prejudice.

Everyone has done their best to support me in their own way and within their own limitations and I am grateful, it is not easy for them. We are all out of our depth with this infection and they don't really know what to do or say. I am never going to get better. On the contrary, I will get progressively sicker.

My needs are suddenly greater than ever before. I am looking for more than people are accustomed to give, perhaps more than they are able to give. People don't welcome change and are slow to adapt. Living on my own I have had to be fairly self-sufficient and, apart from my analysis, I have always tended to be the listener, the comforter, I am not good at expressing my own needs; they are private and will remain so. I just hope that people will be able to perceive them and respond to them; they have their own problems to deal with but at the moment I have enough on my plate without taking on board their worries and depressions too.

People are full of well-meaning advice. I am told constantly to look after myself, keep warm, eat well, take plenty of rest, avoid stress and not to overdo it. These platitudes annoy me and I must learn to accept them in the spirit in which they are intended. I am urged to be positive, told I must have a plan. It is advice which is easily given, but not so easy to interpret and put into practice. They themselves have no ideas or else they forget that I still have the virus and am quite short of funds. I don't have the energy or the money to be travelling around. It is not the opportunity that they imagine it to be. Yes, I will try to be positive and form a plan, but it is more difficult than they realise and I have to be realistic.

For the most part, people seem to have shut their eyes to the full reality of my infection. Perhaps it is too awful to deal with. What I have now is an invisible illness. What they have seen is a reprieve. Now that I look well they can't begin to imagine how it affects me, what I am feeling and experiencing. They don't understand the constant mental anguish and fear.

I am still very thin-skinned and sensitised and seem to have a rather heightened awareness. People hurt me without meaning to and, having nothing very much to occupy myself with I dwell on and magnify the hurt. Why are people blind to themselves? Why do they make no attempt to work themselves out? They look without seeing, listen without hearing. Why can't they see what I see, hear what I hear, share in my perception? It is not they who have changed but I. There has been a split as body and mind have diverged.

I don't really want to be treated very differently from normal. What I want is for people to be kind and pleasant, sensitive to me and my vulnerability and to respect my autonomy. I still need to be given the opportunity to talk about my infection and how I feel. It is not an episode in my life which is now over and can be forgotten; it never will be. I need people's continuing concern and support. And I need to be loved despite the fact that I am homosexual, despite the fact that I have AIDS.

Most of all I crave company and contact with people, I sit for hours, sometimes days, by myself here in my flat and don't see anyone. I run out of ways to occupy myself. A phone call or a cup of coffee with someone makes all the difference, but my friends are all at work and come home tired in the evening and don't want to go out or entertain me.

The two people I was closest to, my father and Howard, are dead. By and large the people I know, apart from Eva, have little unconscious awareness. I am lucky to have her. She is very fond of me and is not involved in the same way my mother and sister are, and I still have Tiger who loves me with all her heart, who is open and intuitive.

It is the people in the clinic who understand best. Dr Kapembwa, Karen, Anne, in fact everyone who works there. They make themselves available for me when I am there and give me the support, encouragement and warmth I need. They are like a family to me.

It is the end of September, the wettest since 1976, and the Autumn colours are exceptionally beautiful this year. The Jag has disappeared from outside; the children are back at school and the squirrels have started hiding their nuts in the lawn. Winter is coming and I know I shall be more vulnerable.

I have ordered my affairs, drawn up my will, arranged for my funeral and sorted out my papers and effects. To my surprise I seem to be reasonably fit and well. There is clearly some life left in me yet and I must turn my attention to making the most of the time I have left; I'm just not quite sure how to go about it, I should be seeking to fulfil my lifetime's ambition, but after forty-two years I don't even know what it is.

I feel the whole of my life has been demolished by one little blood test, but now I must try to rebuild with the bricks which have remained in tact. It's time for me to stop writing, I've said enough and I must try to get on with my life and implement some of my plans, but is it really possible to get on with your life after having been diagnosed as having AIDS or any other life-threatening illness like chronic cancer or leukaemia? It is a death sentence. Most people are not confronted thus brutally with their mortality; they just die. The plans I've made, even the swimming which I so enjoy, just seem like devices to fill in my time until I eventually die and am finally set free from anguish. All there seems left to do is to prepare for death and hope that it will not be too painful or uncomfortable. It is very difficult to think about living in these circumstances.

I may have several years left, though I think it unlikely, but there is a very great sadness which pervades my life and everything I do. The mornings are the worst time for me. I still find it difficult to believe that I have this infection and berate myself for having got into this mess. I feel that nothing really matters anymore and that my life has no point. Then, after the first couple of hours, when the day is underway, my depression lifts and I get on with what I have to do, but the thought of my impending death is always with me and, to an extent, dictates my choices, directs my actions. There is a great urgency to life lest I am overtaken by the infection. When death comes I want to be ready for it. I am more earnest now than ever. Death is a serious business. There is no room in my life for trivial pleasures. I'm frightened to let go and really enjoy myself. I can smile, but laughing is more difficult. My heart isn't in it any more.

It is as though the first cycle of my life is complete and I am about to embark on the last. I am fortunate to have another chance, however short-lived it may be. In a sense there has already been a death. The old life is over and I will never again be quite the same person I was. I wonder what's in store for me now and how long I will have. It is a new beginning, but it is a beginning which embraces an end, the end of my life; it foreshadows my death. It will take courage, fortitude and resolve.

People are getting tired of me and my infection; they don't want the constant worry and anyway it's old news. Life moves on. For me, however, it is a struggle which will go on until I die and it's my fate to bear it.

There is a price to pay, a punishment to be exacted for pursuing what we want, especially if it falls outside normal convention and protocol. After the pleasure there is payment, sometimes retribution. As children we are warned about this in numerous cautionary tales and perhaps we would do well to pay more heed to these stories.

I will not side with the virus or willingly succumb to it. I will continue to fight despite the manifest hopelessness. I may not win the war, but I'll be damned if I can't chalk up a few battles to my credit first. It is not my fault, no matter what people may think. I am not to blame unless we are to attach blame to normal human activities. The drive for sex is very powerful and is intended to find expression. No, I was just unlucky.

This virus is a wicked and dreadful thing. It has already killed hundreds of thousands, if not millions, of people and will probably claim the lives of millions more. I am not a bad person and I don't deserve this. No one does, I feel bitter knowing that I am never going to be wholly well again and that it has affected the last ten years of my life.

I still feel I want to do something or take something which will cure me. The concept of an infection which is incurable is alien. All I can do is remain vigilant, listen to what my body is telling me and look after myself. Much will depend on Dr Kapembwa's skill in treating any infections I get. I am happy to place my trust in him. He is a kind and good man; he is businesslike and skilful. I dream sometimes of miraculous cures; tiny tablets with the name Robert C Gallo imprinted on them and sometimes I dream about dying. After a long, lonely, uphill struggle I am suddenly sitting in a bus bound for paradise, looking out of the window, watching life go on.

It may be that there is nothing I can do to change the course of events and avert the tragedy, but I shall do my best to live with the virus for as long as is possible. The great challenge now is not to let it blight the rest of my life. I will try to make the most of the time I have left. Will I ever give up heart? Never. And if not for my own sake I will try to keep going for Tiger's, fickle though she is. The future is not ours to see; we don't even know what tomorrow will bring. We can only surmise what the future holds.

Man has been searching for answers since human life began. In my way I've been searching too. Maybe the herons know, but I think for us there are no answers. There is no certainty beyond this life. There is only hope, hope that there may be another Spring.

M. D. did in fact see another Spring. However, sadly, he died in February 1995. His writing was finished in 1993.

Appendix 1

Viruses and Retroviruses

Viruses, which are tiny packages of biochemicals, are parasites. They cannot reproduce themselves, nor do they obtain nourishment from the cell they invade. Technically they are non-living. The virus is one hundred times smaller than a bacterium and is measured in millimicrons. It comprises just two substances. The core is nucleic acid and holds the genetic blueprint for producing new virus. This is wrapped in a protective protein cover.

The nucleus of human cells is also nucleic acid. It is DNA (deoxyribonucleic acid). Like the virus it also holds the genetic blueprint in its chromosomes. When cells require a certain protein to fulfil their function they convert a segment of the DNA into RNA (ribonucleic acid). This leaves the nucleus and heads out into the cytoplasm where it sees to the production of protein.

Viruses contain either DNA or RNA, not both. The core of most human viruses is DNA. The virus gets into the cell, takes over the cell's metabolic machinery and tricks it into reading and replicating the viral DNA and producing new virus particles. The cell becomes a virus factory.

There is a small number of viruses which are imprinted in RNA and which affect human beings. They are called retroviruses. Only three have been isolated so far, HTLV-I, HTLV-II (human T-cell lymphotropic viruses) and HIV (human immunodeficiency virus). The first two are responsible for leukaemia and lymphomas, the third is, of course, the AIDS virus. All three attack the T-cells, but whereas HIV destroys them, HTLV-I causes them to proliferate.

The virus locks onto receptor sites on the wall of the cell it chooses to infect. (This is like a plug and socket where the virus is the plug and the cell is the socket.) It enters the cell losing its protein coating.

Having entered the cytoplasm as a strand of RNA it uses a unique enzyme, reverse transcriptase, to convert its RNA into DNA. The new viral DNA, known as the provirus, is so similar to the cell's own DNA that it is received by the nucleus as part of its own DNA and becomes integrated in the cell's chromosomes. Antibodies develop in a couple of months, but most people have no symptoms. It seems to lie dormant for years, but when it takes over, the cell converts the viral DNA into viral RNA producing viral protein and forming new virus particles, known as virions, which emerge from the cell wall at an alarming rate.

Also, through the process of mitosis (cell division) new cells are created. They are identical in every way to the original cell and so, in an AIDS infection, that means the viral DNA and the provirus is propagated in this way.

The HIV virus replicates one hundred times faster than other retroviruses. This is the result of the action of a particular gene within the virus, TAT-III. It produces a protein (the transactivator) which increases replication by up to five thousand fold. This is what makes the virus a killer.

HTLV-I and HTLV-II belong to the retrovirus subfamily of oncoviruses (causing tumours). HIV is a lentivirus (slow acting) because of the length of time between infection and the appearance of symptoms. There are three other known lentiviruses which, in turn, affect sheep, goats and horses. They are so severe and so unresponsive to drugs that the animals have to be slaughtered.

Both the AIDS virus and the other lentiviruses produce neurological impairment since they can infect the brain cells. Seventy per cent of AIDS patients suffer from disorders including depression, delirium and dementia.

Appendix 2

The Immune System

The major components of the immune system are three groups of white blood cells, all of which originate in the bone marrow.

There are the phagocytes, which include the macrophages or 'scavenger' cells. It is their function to engulf and break down viruses, bacteria and cellular debris.

The T-lymphocytes and B-lymphocytes represent the immune system's major resistance to bacteria and viruses that enter the body and cause disease. They are stored in the lymph nodes and spleen.

The B-cells produce thousands of different antibodies. Each B-cell has the ability to make just one type of antibody which is designed to bind onto just one kind of bacterium or virus. Each intruder has its own identifying chemical substances (antigens) on its surface. Some of the B-cells hold on to a 'memory' of the antigen and are ready for it should it appear again.

The T-cells have different functions, but together they control the immune response. The cytotoxic T-cell (killer T-cell) destroys the infected cells. The suppresser T-cell moderates or turns off the immune response by slowing up the B-cells and killer T-cells and halting the body's counterattack when the infection abates. The helper-T (T-4), which is the type the AIDS virus attacks, identifies the antigens of the virus or bacterium and stimulates the B-cells to make antibodies and activates the killer T-cells. The T-4 cell does this by secreting hormone-like substances called lymphokines which serve as a messenger between it, the B-cells and the killer T-cells. The T-4 cell is the most vital member of the immune system. It surveys the body for signs of danger and sets the immune response in motion.

In an AIDS infection the T-4 cells are overwhelmed and the control of the immune system is lost. Antibody production by the B-cells drops and killer cells and macrophages lose their destructive power. The door is open for ordinarily harmless germs to produce sometimes fatal diseases.

Apart from the T-4 cells, the virus also attacks B-cells, macrophages, monocytes, nerve cells and killer T-cells, in fact anything that carries T-4-type receptors on its surface.

Appendix 3

Anti-retroviral Drugs

The majority of anti-HIV drugs work in a similar way, by inhibiting HIV's reverse transcriptase enzyme. This is the case both with the nucleoside analogue drugs such as AZT, ddI and ddC, as well as the non-nucleoside, or alpha-APA compounds, like TIBOL or nevirapine. When HIV infects a cell, it uses reverse transcriptase to make a DNA copy of its genetic information and incorporate it into the cell's chromosomes. If a nucleoside analogue drug is present within the cell, the reverse transcriptase may mistakenly include it when making the copy of the virus's genetic information, effectively sabotaging the process and preventing infection from being completed, Drugs that attack HIV at other points in its lifecycle, such as protease inhibitors and TAT inhibitors are still in the early stages of development.

Some of the side-effect of AZT, such as bone marrow problems leading to shortages of white blood cells (neutropenia) and red blood cells (anaemia), arise because AZT can also inhibit the normal human enzymes which are necessary for cell division (mitosis). Other side-effects are muscle wasting (myopathy), nausea, vomiting and headaches.

ddI and ddC work in a similar way to one another and have similar side-effects and so cannot be used together. They can cause convulsions, diarrhoea, pancreatitis and peripheral neuropathy.

TIBOL (a TIBO-like compound) is an alpha-APA compound or non-nucleoside reverse transcriptase inhibitor. TIBO derivatives are substances related to valium which have been shown to inhibit the replication of HIV (but not other viruses) and to have beneficial effects on surrogate markets such as CD4 counts and p24 viral ant-antigen levels in people with HIV. Early studies with alpha-APA compounds showed that HIV rapidly developed resistance to the drugs meaning that a relatively high dose was required to inhibit those strains of HIV which develop resistance.

Another experimental approach is to use drugs that may stimulate the immune system, such as alpha interferon; it is important that these are combined with anti-virals such as AZT as immune-stimulators may also stimulate HIV replication.

Combination Therapy

HIV is still able to develop resistance to the nucleoside analogue drugs even when they are used in combinations. However, it may be harder for HIV to develop resistance to combinations of anti-HIV drugs as opposed to single drugs used alone. HIV resistance to drugs like AZT and ddI is caused by mutations in the virus's reverse transcriptase gene when it replicates in the presence of the drug.

The development of several different mutations in this gene can also have significant effects. If a person who has developed resistance to AZT switches to ddI, the reverse transcriptase gene may begin to mutate and develop ddI resistance. But the mutations which cause ddI resistance appear, to make the virus susceptible to AZT again. This suggests that if the virus is attacked with the combination of AZT and ddI, the development of resistance will be slowed down.

A similar effect is seen with TIBOL. AZT-resistant HIV becomes susceptible to AZT again after treatment with TIBOL, ddC appears not to prevent the emergence of AZT resistance; however, the effectiveness of the AZT/ddC combination does not seem to be affected even if viral resistance to AZT is present.

Convergent Combination Therapy

It is thought that the development of resistance may be used to improve the effectiveness of treatment. In laboratory tests, a combination of three anti-HIV drugs produced a series of different mutations in the reverse transcriptase enzyme. HIV which developed this series of mutations after exposure to the drug combination appeared to be completely unable to replicate or to infect new cells.

Vaccines

A vaccine is a substance intended to stimulate the body's own immune response against a micro-organism.

A prophylactic vaccine is designed to prevent someone from becoming infected.

A therapeutic vaccine is designed to stimulate the immune response in people who are already infected with the virus.

There are two main types of immune response. One relies on the production of antibodies (humoral immune response). In the case of an HIV infection, the body produces antibodies which lock onto gp120, the viral protein on the surface of the HIV virus. Part of gp120 binds onto the CD4 molecule on the surface of some cells, allowing the virus to infect those cells. By locking onto gp120, these antibodies may prevent the virus from infecting new cells.

The other (cellular immune response) involves the stimulation of T-cells which recognise HIV-infected cells and kills them. However, in HIV, these cytotoxic cells (killer T-cells) seem to disappear from the bloodstream as the illness progresses to AIDS.

When the immune system is activated to respond to an antigen, some of the cells become 'memory' cells. Then, the next time that antigen appears, the immune system is ready to destroy it. This is what is meant by immunity.

Therapeutic vaccines aim to boost the immune response in people who already have an infection. HIV therapeutic vaccines consist of either whole, killed HIV particles, or genetically engineered fragments of the virus.

Surrogate

Surrogate markers are laboratory measurements which seem to predict the likelihood of the development of opportunistic infections or to indicate the extent of damage to the immune system. The most widely used surrogate marker is the CD4 cell count. These are the white blood cells which coordinate the immune system's response to infections. In an HIV infection these cells are progressively depleted.

The count measures the number of cells in a cubic millimetre of blood.

A decline in the number of CD4 cells has been shown to correlate with an increased risk of opportunistic infections and mortality. An increase in the number of cells may indicate a response to anti-HIV treatment.

The CD4 cell count is used to assess the effectiveness of new treatments rather than wait until clinical endpoints, such as opportunistic infections or death, are reached. This enables trials to be completed and effective drugs made available more quickly.

However, HIV is a complicated infection, and the ways in which it harms the immune system are more complex than straightforward depletion of CD4 cells. So a combination of laboratory markers is more reliable than any single laboratory test. Other surrogate markers include: microglobulin, neopterin, p24, anti-HIV vira.